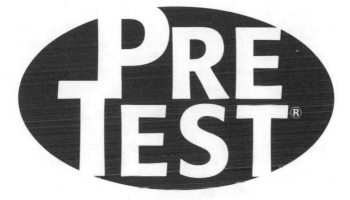

Pediatrics

PreTest® Self-Assessment and Review

NOTICE

Medicine is an ever-changing science. As new research and clinical experience broaden our knowledge, changes in treatment and drug therapy are required. The author and the publisher of this work have checked with sources believed to be reliable in their efforts to provide information that is complete and generally in accord with the standards accepted at the time of publication. However, in view of the possibility of human error or changes in medical sciences, neither the author, nor the publisher, nor any other party who has been involved in the preparation or publication of this work warrants that the information contained herein is in every respect accurate or complete and they disclaim all responsibility for any errors or omissions or for the results obtained from use of the information contained in this work. Readers are encouraged to confirm the information contained herein with other sources. For example and in particular, readers are advised to check the product information sheet included in the package of each drug they plan to administer to be certain that the information contained in this work is accurate and that changes have not been made in the recommended dose or in the contraindications for administration. This recommendation is of particular importance in connection with new or infrequently used drugs.

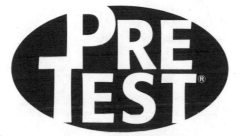

Pediatrics

PreTest® Self-Assessment and Review

Ninth Edition

ROBERT J. YETMAN, M.D.
Professor of Pediatrics
Director, Division of Community and General Pediatrics
University of Texas—Houston Medical School
Houston, Texas

STUDENT REVIEWERS:
Christopher A. Heck
University of South Alabama College of Medicine
Mobile, Alabama

John P. Breinholt III
University of Utah School of Medicine
Salt Lake City, Utah

 McGraw-Hill
Medical Publishing Division
PreTest® Series

NEW YORK   ST. LOUIS   SAN FRANCISCO   AUCKLAND
BOGOTÁ   CARACAS   LISBON   LONDON   MADRID
MEXICO CITY   MILAN   MONTREAL   NEW DELHI
SAN JUAN   SINGAPORE   SYDNEY   TOKYO   TORONTO

McGraw-Hill

A Division of The McGraw·Hill Companies

Pediatrics: PreTest® Self-Assessment and Review, Ninth Edition

Copyright © 2001, 1998, 1995, 1992, 1989, 1987, 1985, 1982, 1978 by The McGraw-Hill Companies, Inc. All rights reserved. Printed in the United States of America. Except as permitted under the Copyright Act of 1976, no part of this publication may be reproduced or distributed in any form or by any means, or stored in a data base or retrieval system, without the prior written permission of the publisher.

2 3 4 5 6 7 8 9 0   DOCDOC   0 1 2

ISBN 0-07-135955-9

This book was set in Berkeley by V&M Graphics.
The editors were Catherine A. Wenz and Karen Davis.
The production supervisor was Richard Ruzycka.
The text designer was Jim Sullivan/Repo Cat Graphics & Editorial Services.
The cover designer was Li Chen Chang/Pinpoint.
R.R. Donnelley & Sons was printer and binder.

This book is printed on acid-free paper.

Library of Congress.Cataloging-in-Publication Data

Pediatrics : PreTest self-assessment and review.—9th ed. / editor, Robert J. Yetman ; student reviewers, Christopher A. Heck, John P. Breinholt III.
    p. ; cm.
    Includes bibliographical references and index.
    ISBN 0-07-135955-9
    1. Pediatrics—Examinations, questions, etc.   I. Yetman, Robert.
    [DNLM: 1. Pediatrics—Examination Questions. WS 18.2 P371 2000]
RJ48.2 .P42 2000
618.92'00076—dc21

00-036143

CONTENTS

INTRODUCTION

Pediatrics: PreTest® Self-Assessment and Review, Ninth Edition, provides comprehensive self-assessment and review within the field of pediatrics. The 500 questions contained in the book have been designed to be similar in format and degree of difficulty to the questions contained in Step 2 of the United States Medical Licensing Examination (USMLE).

Each question has the correct answer, an explanation, and a specific reference to a textbook. A bibliography that lists the sources used in the book follows the last chapter.

Perhaps the most effective way to use this book is to allow yourself one minute to answer each question in a given chapter in order to approximate the time limits imposed by the USMLE Step 2. As you proceed, indicate your answer to each question.

When you have finished answering the questions in a chapter, you should then spend as much time as you need verifying your answers and reading the explanations. Although you should pay special attention to the explanations for the questions you answered incorrectly, you should read every explanation. The editor has designed the explanations to reinforce and supplement the information tested by the questions. If, after reading the explanations, you want more information, you should consult and study the references indicated.

GENERAL PEDIATRICS

Questions

DIRECTIONS: Each item below contains a question or incomplete statement followed by suggested responses. Select the **one best** response to each question.

1. Two weeks after a viral syndrome, a 9-year-old girl presents to your clinic with a complaint of several days of drooping of her mouth. In addition to the drooping of the left side of her mouth, you note that she is unable to completely shut her left eye. Her smile is asymmetric, but her examination is otherwise normal. This girl likely has

a. Guillain-Barré syndrome
b. botulism
c. cerebral vascular accident
d. brainstem tumor
e. Bell's palsy

2. An infant can move his head from side to side while following a moving object, can lift his head from a prone position 45 degrees off the examining table, smiles when encouraged, and makes cooing sounds. He cannot maintain a seated position. The most likely age of the infant is

a. 1 month
b. 3 months
c. 6 months
d. 9 months
e. 12 months

3. A child is brought to your clinic for a routine examine. She can dress with help, ride a tricycle, knows her own age, and can speak in short sentences. She had difficulty in copying a square. The age of this child is most likely

a. 1 year
b. 2 years
c. 3 years
d. 4 years
e. 5 years

4. A 4-year-old girl is noticed by her grandmother to have a limp and a somewhat swollen left knee. The parents report that the patient occasionally complains of pain in that knee. An ophthalmologic examination reveals findings as depicted in the photograph. The condition most likely to be associated with these findings is?

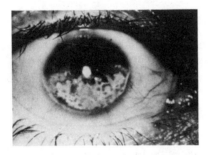

a. juvenile rheumatoid arthritis
b. slipped capital femoral epiphysis
c. Henoch-Schönlein purpura
d. Legg-Calvé-Perthes disease
e. Osgood-Schlatter disease

5. A previously healthy 4-year-old child presents to the emergency room with a 2-day history of a brightly erythematous rash and temperature to 40°C (104°F). The exquisitely tender, generalized rash is worse in the flexural and perioral areas. The child is admitted and over the next day develops crusting and fissuring around the eyes, mouth, and the nose. Sheets of skin tear away with gentle traction. This child most likely has

a. epidermolysis bullosa
b. staphylococcal scalded skin syndrome
c. erythema multiforme
d. drug eruption
e. scarlet fever

6. A scientific study compares two options for the treatment of asthma. The new treatment was found to be statistically superior at the $p < 0.05$ level. This means that

a. the new treatment is 5 percent better than the old treatment
b. a critical threshold for medical significance has been reached
c. 5 percent of the time patients will not benefit from the new therapy
d. the odds are less than 1 in 20 that the differences observed were only a chance variation
e. it would be unethical to continue the old treatment

Items 7–8

7. A previously healthy 8-year-old boy has a 3-week history of low-grade fever of unknown source, fatigue, weight loss, myalgia, and headaches. On repeated examinations during this time, he is found to have a heart murmur, petechiae, and mild splenomegaly. The most likely diagnosis is

a. rheumatic fever
b. Kawasaki disease
c. scarlet fever
d. endocarditis
e. tuberculosis

8. After you make the diagnosis in the previous case, you explain the findings to the family and instruct the family to

a. restrict the child from all strenuous activities
b. give the child a "no salt added" diet
c. ensure that the patient receives antibiotic prophylaxis for dental procedures
d. test all family members in the home
e. avoid allowing the child to get upset

9. A 5-year-old boy who was previously healthy has a 1-day history of low-grade fever, colicky abdominal pain, and a skin rash. He is alert but irritable; temperature is 38.6°C (101.5°F). A diffuse, erythematous, maculopapular and petechial rash is present on his buttocks and lower extremities and shown in the following figure. There is no localized abdominal tenderness or rebound; bowel sounds are active. Laboratory data demonstrate

Urinalysis:	30 red blood cells per high powered field
	2+ protein
Stool:	guaiac positive
Platelet count:	135,000

These findings are most consistent with

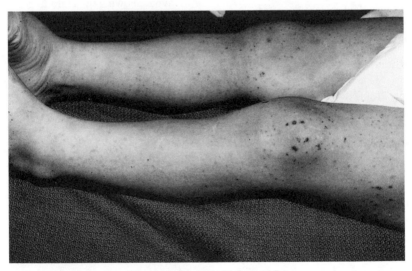

(Courtesy Adelaide Hebert, M.D.)

a. anaphylactoid purpura
b. meningococcemia
c. child abuse
d. leukemia
e. hemophilia B

10. A 4-month-old baby boy has just arrived in the emergency room. He is cold and stiff. History from the parents is that the healthy infant had been placed in his crib for the night and when they next saw him in the morning he was dead. Physical examination is uninformative. Routine whole-body x-rays reveal the abnormality shown. The most likely diagnosis is

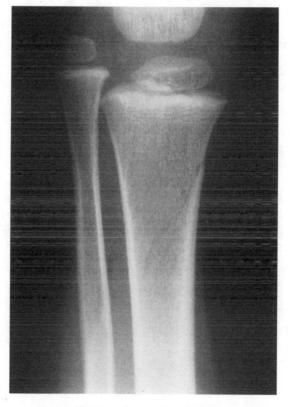

(Courtesy Susan John, M.D.)

a. scurvy
b. congenital syphilis
c. sudden infant death syndrome (SIDS)
d. osteogenesis imperfecta
e. battery

11. A mother brings an 18-month-old to the emergency center with the concern that the child may have ingested a substance. Which of the following is a contraindication to the use of ipecac in this child

a. age less than 5 years
b. breast feeding
c. ingestion of alkali
d. ingestion of iron
e. concurrent administration of intravenous glucose

12. A mother calls you on the telephone and says that her 4-year-old son bit the hand of her 2-year-old son 2 days previously and now the area around the laceration is red, indurated, and swollen and he has a temperature of 103°F (39.4°C). Your immediate response should be to

a. arrange for a plastic surgery consultation to be scheduled in 3 days
b. admit the child to the hospital immediately for surgical debridement and antibiotic treatment
c. prescribe penicillin over the telephone and have the mother apply warm soaks for 15 min qid
d. suggest purchase of bacitracin ointment to apply to the lesion tid
e. see the patient in the emergency room to suture the laceration

Items 13–14

13. A 5-year-old white girl presents with a 14-day history of multiple oval lesions over her back. The rash began with a single lesion over the lower back; the other lesions developed over the next days. These lesions are distributed along the cutaneous cleavage lines and are slightly pruritic. The likely diagnosis is

a. contact dermatitis
b. pityriasis rosea
c. seborrheic dermatitis
d. lichen planus
e. psoriasis

14. The most appropriate initial therapy for the patient in the previous question is

a. phototherapy
b. high-dose topical steroid therapy
c. systemic antifungal agents
d. coal-tar shampoos
e. observation and topical emollients

Items 15–16

15. A very concerned mother brings a 2-year-old child to your office because of multiple episodes of a brief, shrill cry followed by a prolonged expiration and apnea. You have been following this child in your practice since birth and know that the child is a product of a normal pregnancy and delivery, has been growing and developing normally, and has no acute medical problems. The mother relates that the first episode in question occurred immediately after the mother refused to give the child some juice. The child became cyanotic and unconscious and had generalized clonic jerks. A few moments later the child awakened and had no residual effects. A second episode of identical nature occurred at the grocery store when the father of the child refused to purchase a toy for the child. Your physical examination reveals a totally delightful and normal child. The most likely diagnosis in this case is

a.   seizure disorder
b.   drug ingestion
c.   hyperactivity with attention deficit
d.   pervasive development disorder
e.   breath-holding spell

16. The most appropriate course of action in the previous case would be to

a.   obtain an EEG and neurologic consultation prior to starting anticonvulsants
b.   begin anticonvulsants while awaiting the results of an EEG, neurologic consultation, and a urine drug screen
c.   initiate a trial of methylphenidate (Ritalin)
d.   instruct the family to splash cold water on the child's face and begin mouth-to-mouth resuscitation should another episode occur
e.   reassure the family of the likely benign nature of the problem and offer counseling for appropriate behavior modification

17. The 3-day-old infant pictured has a facial rash. The most likely diagnosis is

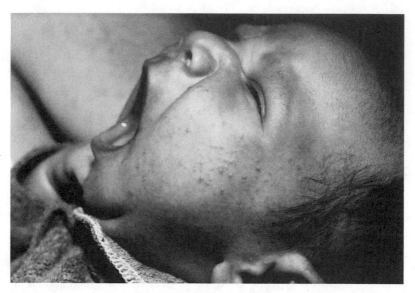

(Courtesy Adelaide Hebert, M.D.)

a. herpes
b. neonatal acne
c. milia
d. seborrheic dermatitis
e. eczema

18. You are called to the emergency room to see one of your patients. The father of this 3-year-old was spraying the yard with an unknown insecticide. In the emergency room, the child is noted to have bradycardia, muscle fasiculations, meiosis, wheezing, and profound drooling. The most likely agent included in this pesticide is

a. organophosphate
b. chlorophenothane (DDT)
c. sodium cyanide
d. warfarin
e. paraquat

19. A 2-year-old child (picture **A**) presents with a four-day history of a rash limited to the feet and ankles. The papular rash is both pruritic and erythematous. The 3-month-old sibling of this patient (picture **B**) has similar lesions also involving the head and neck. Appropriate treatment for this condition includes

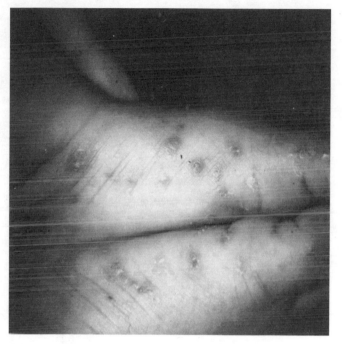

A

a.   local tar soap
b.   permethrin
c.   hydrocortisone cream
d.   emollients
e.   topical antifungal cream

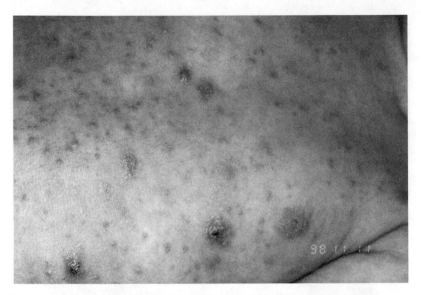

B   (Courtesy Adelaide Hebert, M.D.)

20. An 8-hour-old infant develops increased respiratory distress, hypothermia, and hypotension. A CBC demonstrates a WBC of 2,500 with 80% bands. Which of the following diagnosis is most likely?

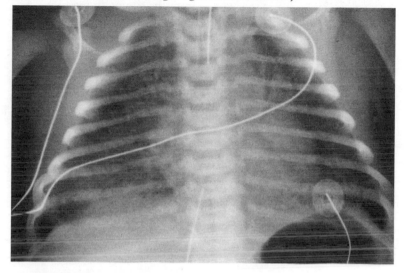

a. gonococcal eye infection
b. diaphragmatic hernia
c. group B streptococcal pneumonia
d. transient tachypnea of the newborn
e. chlamydial pneumonia

21. A 16-year-old basketball player complains of pain in his knees. A physical examination reveals, in addition to tenderness, a swollen and prominent tibial tuberosity. Radiographs of the area are unremarkable. The most likely diagnosis is

a. Osgood-Schlatter disease
b. popliteal cyst
c. slipped capital femoral epiphysis
d. Legg-Calvé-Perthes disease
e. gonococcal arthritis

22. Which of the following statements concerning strabismic amblyopia is true?

a. patching the eye with the greater refractive error is recommended
b. it is prevented if diagnosed before puberty
c. all children should have vision and strabismus screening between ages 5 and 7
d. visual acuity may be restored by prompt treatment at any age
e. central vision may fail to develop if the diagnosis is delayed

23. When counseling a mother of a 2-month-old infant on safety, you tell her that the most common cause of asphyxiation in children is

a. suffocation in old cribs and playpens
b. suffocation in plastic bags
c. inhaling uninflated balloons
d. choking on pacifiers
e. choking on food

24. An infant who sits with only minimal support, attempts to attain a toy beyond reach, and rolls over from the supine to the prone position, but does not have a pincer grasp, is at a developmental level of

a. 2 months
b. 4 months
c. 6 months
d. 9 months
e. 1 year

25. A 5-year-old boy presents with the severe rash pictured as follows. The rash is pruritic and it is especially intense in the flexural areas. The mother reports that the symptoms began in infancy (where it also involved the face) and that her 6-month-old child has similar symptoms. The most likely diagnosis of this condition is

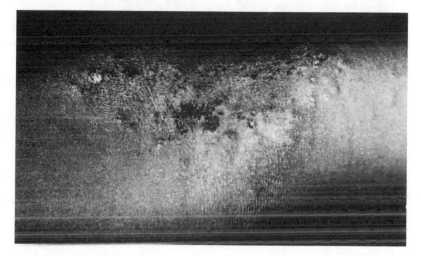

a. seborrheic dermatitis
b. superficial candidiasis
c. psoriasis
d. eczema
e. contact dermatitis

26. Appropriate treatment for the condition described in the previous question includes

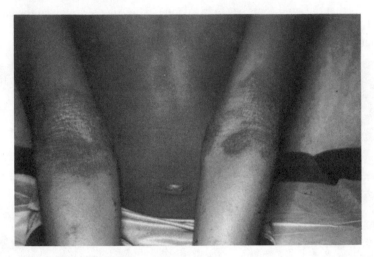

(Courtesy Adelaide Hebert, M.D.)

a.   coal tar soaps and shampoo
b.   topical antifungal cream
c.   ultraviolet light therapy
d.   moisturizers and topical steroids
e.   topical antibiotics

27. An 18-month-old infant has an intensely pruritic scalp with many 0.5-mm translucent eggs noted at the base of hair shafts, especially in the occipital region. The mother of this infant has been using the same hair brush for herself and for her other two children (ages 2 months and 36 months), and a few eggs are noted on each of them. Which of the following therapies should be avoided?

a. treatment of all household contacts with 1% lindane (Kwell)
b. use of 1:1 vinegar:water rinse for hair for nit removal
c. wash all clothing and bedding in very hot water
d. replacement of all commonly used brushes
e. advice to the mother that treatment will again be necessary in 7 to 10 days

28. Thermal injury from immersion in hot water can be prevented by setting water heaters at a temperature no higher than

a. 98.6°F
b. 110°F
c. 120°F
d. 145°F
e. 175°F

29. A 2-year-old boy has been vomiting intermittently for 3 weeks and has been irritable, listless, and anorectic. His use of language has regressed to speaking single words. In your evaluation of this patient, the LEAST likely diagnosis to consider is

a. subdural hematoma
b. brain tumor
c. tuberculous meningitis
d. food allergy
e. lead poisoning

30. Among the following, the LEAST likely risk factor for hearing impairment is

a. a maternal history of use of phenytoin during pregnancy
b. a family history of hearing impairment
c. craniofacial abnormalities
d. birth weight less than 1500 g
e. neonatal hyperbilirubinemia

Items 31–32

31. An 8-month-old infant has a 2-day history of diarrhea and poor fluid intake. You diagnose a 10 percent to 15 percent dehydration. Which of the following fluids is appropriate to begin immediate resuscitation?

a. D_5 ¼ normal saline
b. D_5 ½ normal saline
c. normal saline
d. whole blood
e. $D_{10}W$

32. In this patient, you decide to give 20 mL per kilogram of the chosen fluid. A reasonable period of time over which to infuse this fluid is

a. 2.5 min
b. 60 min
c. 4 h
d. 8 h
e. 24 h

33. A systolic blood pressure of 120 mm Hg is normal for children above age

a. 1 year
b. 4 years
c. 7 years
d. 10 years
e. 12 years

34. A 20-month-old child is brought to the emergency department because of fever and irritability and refusal to move his right lower extremity. Physical examination reveals a swollen and tender right knee that resists passive motion. The most important test to confirm the impression of septic arthritis is

a. examination of joint fluid
b. x-ray of the knee
c. erythrocyte sedimentation rate (ESR)
d. complete blood count (CBC) and differential
e. blood culture

35. A 15-year-old high school boy sustained an abrasion of the knee after a fall while roller blading in the school yard. School records reveal that his last DPT booster was at age 6. In this situation, which of the following is appropriate?

a. tetanus toxoid
b. adult tetanus and diphtheria toxoid (Td)
c. DPT booster
d. tetanus toxoid and tetanus immune globulin
e. no immunization

36. There are over 1 million emergency room visits each year in the United States for mammalian bites. In addition to consideration of tetanus and rabies prophylaxis for these bites, the question of antibiotic prophylaxis is of concern. Indications for antibiotic prophylaxis include which of the following

a. the wound cannot be adequately debrided
b. the wound is a dog bite
c. primary closure is planned
d. the bite is on the abdomen
e. the victim is an 18-month-old toddler

37. Aunt Mary is helping her family move to a new apartment. During the confusion, 3-year-old Jimmy is noted to be stumbling about, his face flushed, and his speech slurred. The contents of Aunt Mary's purse are strewn about on the floor. In the emergency room, Jimmy is found to have a rapid heart beat, blood pressure of 42/20, and dilated pupils. ECG shows prolonged QRS and QT intervals. Jimmy suddenly starts to convulse. His condition is most likely to be the result of poisoning with

a. barbiturates
b. tricyclic antidepressants
c. diazepam
d. organophosphates
e. arsenic

38. As a city public health officer you have been charged with the task of screening children for lead poisoning. The best screen for this purpose is

a. careful physical examination of each infant and child
b. erythrocyte protoporphyrin levels (EP, FEP, or ZPP)
c. CBC and blood smear
d. blood lead level
e. environmental history

39. Universal immunization of infants with a three-dose series of intramuscular, genetically engineered hepatitis B surface antigen vaccine is recommended. Implementation of this recommendation should decrease the incidence of which of the following

a. neonatal hyperbilirubinemia
b. alcoholic liver disease
c. Dubin-Johnson syndrome
d. hepatocellular carcinoma
e. hydrops of the gallbladder

40. New parents ask you how to reduce the chance of their baby suffering from sudden infant death syndrome (SIDS). You tell them to place the child in which of the following for sleep

a. supine position
b. prone position
c. seated position
d. Trendelenburg position
e. a hammock

41. A mentally retarded 14-year-old boy has a long face, large ears, micropenis, and large testes. Chromosome analysis is likely to demonstrate which of the following

a. trisomy 21
b. trisomy 18
c. trisomy 13
d. fragile X syndrome
e. William's syndrome

42. "Normal," or "physiologic," saline has which of the following characteristics

a. Na^+ 154 mEq/L and Cl^- 154 mEq/L
b. 0.9 g of NaCl in 1 L of water
c. 10 g of dextrose in 1 L of water
d. physiologic ratio of Na^+ to Cl^-
e. 28 mEq of lactate per L

DIRECTIONS: Each group of questions below consists of lettered options followed by numbered items. For each numbered item, select the appropriate lettered option(s). Each lettered option may be used once, more than once, or not at all. **Choose exactly the number of options indicated following each item.**

Items 43–48

Many rashes and skin lesions can be found in the newborn period. For each of the descriptions listed below, select the most likely diagnosis.

a. sebaceous nevi
b. salmon patch
c. neonatal acne
d. pustular melanosis

e. erythema toxicum
f. seborrheic dermatitis
g. milia

43. Examination of fluid from this lesion demonstrates eosinophils **(SELECT 1 DIAGNOSIS)**

44. Frequently found over the eyelids, glabella, and nape of neck, this lesion fades over the first weeks of life **(SELECT 1 DIAGNOSIS)**

45. Resolution of this lesion results in a hyperpigmented spot, which resolves over several days **(SELECT 1 DIAGNOSIS)**

46. Usually identified as a yellowish, hair-free lesion on the scalp; this lesion is potentially premalignant **(SELECT 1 DIAGNOSIS)**

47. Fine, white, 1- to 2-mm lesions scattered over the face and gingivae of the neonate **(SELECT 1 DIAGNOSIS)**

48. Frequently presents as cradle cap in the newborn period **(SELECT 1 DIAGNOSIS)**

Items 49–53

An understanding of the pathogenesis of the various diseases for which an active immunization is available leads to an appreciation of the nature of the immunizing material. For each of the diseases listed below, select the appropriate active immunizing material.

a. intramuscular mutant toxin
b. intramuscular polysaccharide with protein adjuvant
c. intramuscular toxoid
d. oral attenuated live virus
e. subcutaneous attenuated live virus
f. intramuscular whole killed bacilli

49. Diphtheria **(SELECT 1 SUBSTANCE)**

50. Tetanus **(SELECT 1 SUBSTANCE)**

51. *Haemophilus influenzae* type b **(SELECT 1 SUBSTANCE)**

52. Measles **(SELECT 1 SUBSTANCE)**

53. Rubella **(SELECT 1 SUBSTANCE)**

Items 54–58

For each of the injuries listed below, select the age at which it is most likely to occur.

a. 6 months
b. 1 year
c. 2 years
d. 6 years
e. 10 years

54. Asphyxiation and choking **(SELECT 1 AGE)**

55. Drowning in swimming pools **(SELECT 1 AGE)**

56. Pedestrian injury **(SELECT 1 AGE)**

57. Baby-walker injuries **(SELECT 1 AGE)**

58. Accidental poisoning **(SELECT 1 AGE)**

Items 59–62

For each disorder below, select the dietary deficiency that is likely to be responsible.

a. caloric deficiency
b. thiamine deficiency
c. niacin deficiency
d. vitamin D deficiency
e. vitamin C deficiency
f. vitamin B_{12} deficiency
g. vitamin B_6 deficiency
h. biotin deficiency
i. riboflavin deficiency

59. Progressive weight loss, constipation, muscular atrophy, loss of skin turgor, hypothermia, and edema **(SELECT 1 DEFICIENCY)**

60. Dermatitis, diarrhea, and dementia **(SELECT 1 DEFICIENCY)**

61. Congestive heart failure, peripheral neuritis, and psychic disturbances **(SELECT 1 DEFICIENCY)**

62. Enlargement of costochondral junction, craniotabes, and scoliosis **(SELECT 1 DEFICIENCY)**

Items 63–66

For each of the syndromes below that can cause childhood deafness, select the clinical finding with which it is most likely to be associated.

a. pulmonary stenosis
b. white forelock
c. goiter
d. retinitis pigmentosa
e. polydactyly

63. Waardenburg syndrome b
(SELECT 1 FINDING)

64. Pendred's syndrome c
(SELECT 1 FINDING)

65. Usher's syndrome d
(SELECT 1 FINDING)

66. LEOPARD syndrome a
(SELECT 1 FINDING)

Items 67–70

For each disorder listed below, select the gender and age distribution with which it is most likely to be associated.

a.   males 2 to 12 years of age
b.   males 9 to 15 years of age
c.   females 4 to 10 years of age
d.   females 11 to 16 years of age
e.   females and males 1 to 4 years of age

67. Legg-Calvé-Perthes disease **(SELECT 1 GROUP)**

68. Slipped capital femoral epiphysis **(SELECT 1 GROUP)**

69. Progressive idiopathic scoliosis requiring treatment **(SELECT 1 GROUP)**

70. Subluxation of the head of the radius (nursemaid's elbow) **(SELECT 1 GROUP)**

Items 71–75

For poisoning by each substance below, match the appropriate treatment.

a.   atropine and pralidoxime (2-PAM)
b.   N-Acetylcysteine (Mucomyst)
c.   Meso-2,3-dimercaptosuccimic acid (DMSA succimer)
d.   naloxone (Narcan)
e.   sodium bicarbonate

71. Lead **(SELECT 1 TREATMENT)**

72. Acetaminophen **(SELECT 1 TREATMENT)**

73. Morphine **(SELECT 1 TREATMENT)**

74. Salicylate **(SELECT 1 TREATMENT)**

75. Organophosphate insecticide **(SELECT 1 TREATMENT)**

Items 76–78

For poisoning by each substance below, match the treatment indicated.

a. deferoxamine mesylate
b. diphenhydramine (Benadryl)
c. acetazolamide and sodium bicarbonate
d. ethanol
e. dimercaprol (BAL)

76. Phenothiazine **(SELECT 1 TREATMENT)**

77. Iron **(SELECT 1 TREATMENT)**

78. Methanol **(SELECT 1 TREATMENT)**

Items 79–83

Excess vitamin intake has been shown to have deleterious effects. Match the vitamin with the toxic effect.

a. kidney stones
b. sensory neuropathy
c. edema
d. hyperostosis ↑ bone growth
e. calcification of the heart
f. decreased cerebrospinal fluid pressure
g. erythema of skin

79. Vitamin A **(SELECT 1 EFFECT)**

80. Nicotinic acid **(SELECT 1 EFFECT)**

81. Vitamin C **(SELECT 1 EFFECT)**

82. Vitamin D **(SELECT 1 EFFECT)**

83. Pyridoxine **(SELECT 1 EFFECT)**

Items 84–88

The normal development of the fetus can be adversely affected by exposure to a number of environmental factors, including infectious agents, physical agents, chemical agents, and maternal metabolic and genetic agents. Match each teratogen with the most likely clinical presentation.

a. small palpebral fissures, ptosis, midfacial hypoplasia, smooth philtrum
b. hypoplasia of distal phalanges, small nails
c. bilateral microtia or anotia
d. spina bifida
e. heart block
f. sacral agenesis
g. aniridia
h. hemangiomatosis

84. Maternal diabetes **(SELECT 1 PRESENTATION)**

85. Phenytoin **(SELECT 1 PRESENTATION)**

86. Valproate **(SELECT 1 PRESENTATION)**

87. Alcohol **(SELECT 1 PRESENTATION)**

88. Maternal lupus erythematosus **(SELECT 1 PRESENTATION)**

Items 89–92

Match each common skin condition with the most appropriate therapy.

a. mild cleansing cream, topical moisturizers, and topical steroids
b. topical or oral antibacterial agents
c. oral antihistamines alone
d. brief application of liquid nitrogen, cantharidin 0.9%, or extrusion of lesion's central plug with curette
e. permethrin 5% cream (Elimite)
f. topical acyclovir
g. topical antifungal agents

89. Impetigo **(SELECT 1 TREATMENT)**

90. Scabies **(SELECT 1 TREATMENT)**

91. Molluscum contagiosum **(SELECT 1 TREATMENT)**

92. Atopic dermatitis **(SELECT 1 TREATMENT)**

Items 93–95

Heart failure is possible at any age. Match each clinical condition with the most likely diagnosis.

a.   glomerulonephritis
b.   severe anemia
c.   heart block
d.   ventricular septal defect
e.   arteriovenous malformation
f.   coarctation of the aorta

93. A 6-month-old child with a loud systolic murmur at the left lower sternal border **(SELECT 1 DIAGNOSIS)**

94. A 14-year-old child with headache, hypertension, edema, and a change in urine output and color **(SELECT 1 DIAGNOSIS)**

95. A 3-day-old infant born to a mother with active systemic lupus erythematosus (SLE) **(SELECT 1 DIAGNOSIS)**

Items 96–102

The Committee on Nutrition of the American Academy of Pediatrics has concluded that children on a normal diet do not need vitamin supplements. There are, however, some clinical situations in infancy and childhood in which special needs do occur. Match each situation with the appropriate supplement.

a. all fat-soluble vitamins   d. vitamin D
b. pyridoxine   e. vitamin K
c. vitamin A   f. folate

96. Isoniazid therapy **(SELECT 1 SUPPLEMENT)**

97. Administration of phenytoin **(SELECT 1 SUPPLEMENT)**

98. Measles in developing countries **(SELECT 1 SUPPLEMENT)**

99. Liver disease **(SELECT 1 SUPPLEMENT)**

100. Breast-fed infant **(SELECT 1 SUPPLEMENT)**

101. Sickle cell disease **(SELECT 1 SUPPLEMENT)**

102. One-day-old newborn **(SE-LECT 1 SUPPLEMENT)**

Items 103–107

Match each clinical condition with the appropriate diagnostic laboratory test.

a. erythrocyte sedimentation rate
b. serum immunoglobulin levels
c. nitroblue tetrazolium (NBT) test
d. CH50 assay
e. CBC demonstrating Howell-Jolly bodies
f. platelet count
g. intradermal skin test using *Candida albicans*

103. Phagocytic-cell defects **(SELECT 1 TEST)**

104. Wiskott-Aldrich syndrome **(SELECT 1 TEST)**

105. B-cell defect **(SELECT 1 TEST)**

106. T-cell defect **(SELECT 1 TEST)**

107. Asplenia **(SELECT 1 TEST)**

GENERAL PEDIATRICS

Answers

1. The answer is e. (*Behrman, 16/e, p. 1893. McMillan, 3/e, p. 1963. Rudolph, 20/e, p. 2074.*) Bell's palsy is an acute, unilateral facial nerve palsy that begins about 2 weeks after a viral infection. The exact pathophysiology is unknown but it is thought to be immune or allergic. On the affected side, the upper and lower face are typically, paretic, the mouth droops, and the patient cannot close the eye. Treatment consists of maintaining moisture to the affected eye (especially at night) to prevent keratitis. Complete, spontaneous resolution occurs in about 85 percent of cases, 10 percent of cases have mild residual disease, and about 5 percent of cases do not resolve.

2. The answer is b. (*Behrman, 15/e, p. 35. McMillan, 3/e, pp. 756–761. Rudolph, 21/e, pp. 121–128.*) Infants who are developing normally should be able to smile and coo when smiled at or talked to by 8 weeks of age. By 3 months of age, infants should be able to follow a moving toy not only from side to side but also in the vertical plane. When placed on his or her abdomen, a normal 3-month-old infant can raise his or her face 45° to 90° from the horizontal. Not until 6 to 8 months of age should an infant be able to maintain a seated position.

3. The answer is c. (*Behrman, 16/e, p. 38. McMillan, 3/e. pp. 756–761. Rudolph, 20/e, pp. 121–128.*) By 3 years of age, children become quite skilled in many areas. Most can say many words and speak in sentences. They can help dress and undress themselves with the exception of shoelaces and sometimes, buttons. They can ride a tricycle and can alternate feet when climbing stairs, although they still place both feet on each step when going down stairs. They can identify at least one color by name, know their age and gender, but have not progressed beyond copying a circle and a crude cross. Only at 4 to 5 years of age can a child copy a square.

4. The answer is a. (*Behrman, 16/e, pp. 704–709. McMillan, 3/e, pp. 2156–2160. Rudolph, 2/e, pp. 479–483.*) Pauciarticular rheumatoid arthritis asymmetrically involves large joints, especially the knee, and often has no other symptoms. The major morbidity of pauciarticular rheumatoid arthritis is blindness. About 20 percent of girls who have the monoarthritic or pauciarticular form of juvenile rheumatoid arthritis have iridocyclitis as their only significant systemic manifestation. Because this eye disorder can require treatment with local or systemic steroids and develop without signs or symptoms, it is recommended that all children with this form of arthritis have frequent slit-lamp eye examinations.

5. The answer is b. (*Behrman, 16/e, pp. 2031. McMillan, 3/e, pp. 378–379, 418–420. Rudolph, 20/e, p. 930.*) Also known as Ritter disease, staphylococcal scalded skin disease is seen most commonly in children less than 5 years of age. The rash is preceded by fever, irritability, and erythema and extraordinary tenderness of the skin. Circumoral erythema; crusting of the eyes, mouth, and nose; and blisters on the skin can develop. Intraoral mucosal surfaces are not affected. Peeling of the epidermis in response to mild shearing forces (Nikolsky sign) leaves the patient susceptible to problems similar to those of a burn injury, including infection and fluid and electrolyte imbalance. Cultures of the bullae are negative but the source site is often positive. Treatment includes antibiotics (to cover resistant *Staphylococcus aureus*) and localized skin care. Recovery without scarring can be expected.

6. The answer is d. (*McMillan, 3/e, pp. 38–39.*) The probability given is an estimation of the odds that the observed differences could have occurred by chance alone. The interpretation of these results depends on an assessment of factors such as study design, the size of the sample, the type of controls used, the severity of the disease, the side effects, and the importance of the treatment. The tendency for negative results to remain unpublished should also be kept in mind.

7–8. The answers are 7–d, 8–c. (*Behrman, 16/e, pp. 1424–1428. McMillan, 3/e, pp. 1405–1417. Rudolph, 20/e, pp. 1522–1526.*) The presentation of infective endocarditis can be quite variable, ranging from prolonged fever with few other symptoms to an acute and severe course with early toxicity. A high index of suspicion is necessary to make the diagnosis quickly. Identification of the causative organism (frequently *Streptococcus* sp. or *Staphylococcus* sp.) through multiple blood cultures is imperative for appropriate treatment. Echocardiography may identify valvular vegetations and can be predictive of impending embolic events. Treatment usually consists of 4 to 6 weeks of appropriate antimicrobial therapy. Bed rest should only be instituted for heart failure. Antimicrobial prophylaxis prior to and after dental cleaning is indicated.

9. The answer is a. (*Behrman, 16/e, pp. 728–729. McMillan, 3/e, pp. 1490–1491, 2176–2179. Rudolph, 20/e, pp. 497, 910, 1240–1241, 1359.*) The clinical presentation described supports the diagnosis of anaphylactoid purpura, a generalized, acute vasculitis of unknown cause involving small blood vessels. In this condition, the skin lesion, which is classic in character and distribution, is often accompanied by arthritis, usually of the large joints, and by gastrointestinal symptoms. Colicky abdominal pain, vomiting, and melena are common. Renal involvement occurs in a significant number of patients and is potentially the most serious manifestation of the disease. Although most children with this complication recover, some will develop chronic nephritis. Laboratory studies are not diagnostic. Serum complement and IgA levels can be normal or elevated. Coagulation studies and platelets are normal.

10. The answer is e. (*Behrman, 16/e, pp. 110–114. McMillan, 3/e, pp. 507–524. Rudolph, 20/e, pp. 145–151.*) The x-ray showing a fracture (or an x-ray showing multiple fractures in various stages of healing) indicates trauma. This information should be reported to the medical examiner and appropriate social agencies, including the police, so that an investigation can be started and other children in the home or under the care of the same babysitter can be protected. Although an autopsy (and death-scene investigation) should be done in every such case, there sometimes develops a tendency for medical examiners to diagnose SIDS without an autopsy, particularly if the parents object to one, unless further information is provided by the emergency room staff as in this case.

11. The answer is c. (*Behrman 16/e, p. 2226. McMillan, 3/e, pp. 618–619. Rudolph, 20/e, p. 815.*) The induction of emesis by the use of syrup of ipecac is a very effective method of removing swallowed poisons. It has been used safely in children as young as 6 months of age. Ipecac should not be given to a patient who has ingested a corrosive poison, such as strong acid or alkali, because of the possibility of gastric perforation and further necrosis of the esophagus. When vomiting imposes a risk of aspiration, as in the case of an obtunded or comatose patient or in the case of impending seizures precipitated by the ingested drug, syrup of ipecac is contraindicated. Hydrocarbons such as mineral oil have a low viscosity and surface tension; the latter property accounts for the spreading tendency of the product and the potential for aspiration. Very minute amounts of aspirated hydrocarbon can cause a necrotizing pneumonia. Syrup of ipecac should be used only when the primary toxicity of the hydrocarbon is systemic, as for example, with carbon tetrachloride or benzene. Administration of activated charcoal alone without prior gut emptying is being used for certain ingestions. Proper instruction of parents regarding toxic ingestions should be provided during well-child visits. Efforts should be aimed at prevention, with age-appropriate anticipatory guidance regarding environmental hazards.

12. The answer is b. (*Behrman, 16/e, pp. 790–792. McMillan, 3/e, pp. 587–589.*) Human bites can pose a significant problem. They can become infected with oropharyngeal bacteria, including *Staphylococcus aureus*, viridans streptococci, *Bacteroides* species, and anaerobes. A patient with an infected human bite of the hand requires hospitalization for appropriate drainage procedures; Gram stain and culture of the exudate, vigorous cleaning, debridement, and appropriate antibiotics. The wound should be left open and allowed to heal by secondary intention.

13–14. The answers are 13–b, 14–e. (*Behrman, 16/e, pp. 2001–2007. McMillan, 3/e, pp. 689, 720. Rudolph, 20/e, p. 894.*) Pityriasis rosea is a benign condition that usually presents with a herald patch, a single round or oval lesion appearing anywhere on the body. Usually about 5 to 10 days after the appearance of the herald patch, a more diffuse rash involving the upper extremities and trunk appears. These lesions are oval or round, slightly raised, and pink to brown in color. The lesion is covered in a fine scale with some central clearing possible. The rash can appear in the Christmas tree pattern on the back identified by the aligning of the long axis of the lesions with the cutaneous cleavage lines. The rash lasts 2 to 12 weeks and can be pruritic. This rash is commonly mistaken for tinea corporis, and the consideration of secondary syphilis is important.

Treatment is usually unnecessary but can consist of topical emollients and oral antihistamines as needed. More uncommonly, topical steroids can be helpful if the itching is severe.

Lichen planus is rare in children. It is intensely pruritic and additional lesions can be induced with scratching. The lesion is commonly found on the flexor surfaces of the wrists, forearms, inner thighs, and occasionally on the oral mucosa.

Seborrheic dermatitis can begin anytime during life; it frequently presents as cradle cap in the newborn period. This rash is commonly greasy, scaly, and erythematous and in smaller children, involves the face, neck, axilla, and diaper area. In older children, the rash can be localized to the scalp and intertriginous areas. Pruritus can be marked.

Contact dermatitis is characterized by redness, weeping, and oozing of the affected skin. The pattern of distribution can be helpful in identification of the offending agent. The rash can be pruritic; removal of the causative agent and use of topical emollients or steroids is curative.

Psoriasis consists of red papules that coalesce to form plaques with sharp edges. A thick, silvery scale develops on the surface and leaves a drop of blood upon its removal (Auspitz's sign). Additional lesions develop upon scratching older lesions. Commonly affected sites include scalp, knees, elbows, umbilicus, and genitalia.

15–16. The answers are 15–e, 16–e. *(Behrman, 16/e, pp. 1829–1830. Rudolph 20/e p. 128.)* The child in this question most likely has breath-holding spells. Two forms exist. Cyanotic spells consist of the symptoms outlined and are predictable upon upsetting or scolding the child. They are rare before 6 months of age, peak at about 2 years of age, and resolve by about 5 years of age. Avoidance of reinforcing this behavior is the treatment of choice. Pallid breath-holding spells are less common and are usually caused by a painful experience (such as a fall). With these events, the child will stop breathing, lose consciousness, become pale and hypotonic, and may have a brief tonic episode. These, too, resolve spontaneously. Again, avoidance of reinforcing behavior is indicated.

17. The answer is b. *(Behrman, 16/e, pp. 2044–2050. McMillan, 3/e, pp. 684, 730. Rudolph, 20/3, p. 925.)* The pictured infant has a classic case of neonatal acne, which peaks at 2 to 4 weeks of age. The condition results from maternal hormone transmission. It resolves in a few weeks to months, and occasionally is severe enough to require treatment with agents such as 2.5% benzoyl peroxide.

18. The answer is a. *(Behrman, 16/e, pp. 2152–2153, 2162. McMillan, 3/e, p. 621. Rudolph, 20/e, pp. 842–843.)* When the clinical signs of constricted pupils, bradycardia, and muscle fasciculations are associated with the sudden onset of neurologic symptoms, progressive respiratory distress, diaphoresis, diarrhea, and overabundant salivation, a diagnosis of organophosphate poisoning should be suspected. Intake of organophosphate agents can occur by ingestion, inhalation, or absorption through skin or mucosa. Organophosphates inhibit carboxylic esterase enzymes, including acetylcholinesterase and pseudocholinesterase; toxicity depends primarily on the inactivation or inhibition of acetylcholinesterase. Treatment consists of gastric lavage, if the poison has been ingested, or decontamination of the skin, if exposure has been through contact. Maintenance of adequate ventilation and fluid and electrolyte balance also is indicated. All symptomatic children should receive atropine and, if severely affected, cholinesterase-reactivating oximes as well. Cholinesterase-reactivating oximes quickly restore consciousness by inhibiting muscarine- and nicotine-like synaptic actions of acetylcholine. Cholinesterase-reactivating oximes include pralidoxime chloride or obidoxime.

19. The answer is b. *(Behrman, 16/e, pp. 2044–2046. McMillan, 3/e, pp. 716–717. Rudolph, 20/e, pp. 780–781.)* Scabies is caused by the mite *Sarcoptes scabiei* var. *hominis*. Most older children and adults present with intensely pruritic and threadlike burrows in the interdigital areas, groin, elbows, and ankles; the palms, soles, face, and head are spared. Infants, however, usually present with bullae and pustules and the areas spared in adults are often involved in infants. The clinical manifestations closely resemble those of atopic dermatitis. Because of the potential neurotoxic effect to infants of gamma benzene hexachloride through percutaneous absorption, an excellent alternative—5% permethrin cream (Elimite)—is available and is more often recommended.

20. The answer is c. *(Behrman, 16/e, pp. 810–816. McMillan, 3/e, pp. 421–427. Rudolph, 20/e, pp. 1607–1608.)* The rapid onset of the symptoms, the low WBC count with left shift, and the depicted chest x-ray findings are typical of a patient with group B streptococcus pneumonia. Appropriate management would include rapid recognition of symptoms, respiratory support, and rapid institution of appropriate antibiotics. Despite these measures, mortality from this infection is not uncommon. The other infectious causes listed do not present so early, and the noninfectious causes listed do not cause elevations in the band count.

21. The answer is a. (*Behrman, 15/e, pp. 2075–2076, 2080–2082, 2106. McMillan, 3/e, pp. 749, 2109–2110. Rudolph 20/e, p. 2148.*) This history is typical of Osgood-Schlatter disease. Microfractures in the area of the insertion of the patellar tendon into the tibial tubercle are common in athletic adolescents. Swelling, tenderness, and an increase in size of the tibial tuberosity are found. Radiographs can be necessary to rule out other conditions. Treatment consists of rest.

Legg-Calvé-Perthes disease is avascular necrosis of the femoral head. This condition usually produces mild or intermittent pain in the anterior thigh but can also present as a painless limp.

Gonococcal arthritis, although common in this age range, is uncommon in this anatomic site. More significant systemic signs and symptoms, including chills, fever, migratory polyarthralgias, and rash, are commonly seen.

Slipped capital femoral epiphysis is usually seen in a younger, more obese child (mean age about 10 years) or in the thinner, older child who has just undergone a rapid growth spurt. Pain upon movement of the hip is diagnostic.

Popliteal cysts are found on the posterior aspect of the knee.

22. The answer is e. (*Behrman, 16/e, pp. 587, 2106, 2106. McMillan, 3/e, p. 672. Rudolph, 20/e, pp. 2065, 2111, 2121–2122.*) To prevent monocular blindness and to assure the development of normal binocular vision, early recognition and treatment of strabismus are essential. Infants can be screened for strabismus by observing the location of a light reflection in the pupils when the patient fixes on a light source. Normally, it should be in the center or just nasal of the center in each pupil. Persistence of a transient or fixed deviation of an eye beyond 4 months of age requires referral to an ophthalmologist. The aim of treatment is to prevent loss of central vision from foveal suppression of a confusing image in the deviating eye. This is accomplished by surgery, eyeglasses, or patching of the normal eye. The prognosis for normal vision if diagnosis is delayed beyond 6 years of age is guarded. Routine vision and strabismus screening is essential at age 3 to 4 years.

23. The answer is e. (*Behrman, 16/e, pp. 231, 1279–1280. McMillan, 3/e, p. 500.*) Childhood fatalities from asphyxiation are concentrated among children younger than 4. The most common cause of asphyxiation is choking on foods of the size, shape, and consistency to occlude the upper airway completely. Foods that are particularly dangerous include round hard candies, hot dogs, whole grapes, and pieces of raw apple or carrot. Children are also at risk of aspirating small objects like round, pliable toys, uninflated balloons, makeshift pacifiers, bottle nipples, and plastic-lined disposable diapers. Asphyxiation can also occur from external compression of the airway, as can occur in defective cribs or playpens. Cribs manufactured since 1974 comply with regulations for slat spacing of 2⅜ inches or less.

24. The answer is c. (*Behrman, 16/e, pp. 35–37. McMillan, 3/e, pp. 756–761. Rudolph, 20/e, pp. 121–128.*) At 6 to 6½ months of age, infants will be able to sit alone, leaning forward to support themselves with arms extended, the so-called tripod position. They can reach for an object by changing the orientation of the torso. They can purposefully roll from a prone to supine as well as from a supine to prone position. By 12 months, they can grasp a pellet between thumb and forefinger without ulnar support. Motor development occurs in a cephalocaudal and central-to-peripheral direction. Therefore, truncal control precedes arm control, which precedes finger dexterity.

25–26. The answers are 25–d, 26–d. (*Behrman 16/e, pp. 680–684. McMillan, 3/e, pp. 704–706. Rudolph, 20/e, pp. 889–892.*) Eczema is a chronic dermatitis that occurs in a population with a strong personal or family history of atopy. The skin presents initially as an erythematous, papulovesicular, weeping eruption, which progresses over time to a scaly, lichenified dermatitis. From 3 months to 2 years of age, the rash is prominent on the cheeks, wrists, scalp, postauricular areas, and arms and legs. In the young child 2 to 12 years of age, the extensor surfaces of arms, legs, and neck are mainly involved. Pruritus is a predominant feature, and scratching leads to excoriation, secondary infection, and lichenification of the skin. The rash has a chronic and relapsing course and treatment is determined by the major clinical features. Cutaneous irritants (bathing in hot water, scrubbing vigorously with soap, wearing wool or synthetic clothing) should be avoided, and maximal skin hydration with emollients is essential. Topical moisturizers and steroids are the mainstays of therapy for atopic dermatitis. The use of antihistamines can provide additional relief from pruritus.

27. The answer is a. *(Behrman, 16/e, pp. 2046–2047. McMillan, 3/e, p. 716. Rudolph 20/e, pp. 783, 936.)* All the treatments outlined for this patient with head lice *(Pediculosis capitis)* are appropriate except for use of 1% lindane in small infants. The treatment of choice for these small children is permethrin 1% cream rinse (Nix).

28. The answer is c. *(Behrman 16/e, p. 235. McMillan, 3/e, pp. 499–500. Rudolph, 20/e, p. 28.)* Significant morbidity from immersion in hot water can be prevented by setting the temperature of water heaters at 120°F. A third-degree burn can result from immersion in water at a temperature greater than 130°F for less than 5 sec. Immersion burns that are the result of intentional injury are seen most frequently in children between the ages of 1 and 3 years, the period during which toilet training is in progress. Careful examination of the location, distribution, and depth of the burn will provide clues as to the position of the child during the immersion. The injured child should be examined thoroughly for other signs of neglect and abuse

29. The answer is d. *(Behrman 16/e pp. 653–654, 890–891, 1859, 2107, 2156–2159. McMillan, 3/e, pp. 615–616, 632, 1033, 1511–1512, 1689–1692. Rudolph, 20/e, pp. 618, 835–837, 1900–1905, 1936.)* Unfortunately, the seriousness of the illness in a child such as this will often be unrecognized, and the patient will be diagnosed as having an incipient nondisease and treated symptomatically. Although it is true that many patients with non-specific complaints have trivial diseases that resolve spontaneously, the patient presented here has a 3-week history with potentially grave implications. Diagnoses other than food allergy should be considered foremost.

30. The answer is a. *(Behrman, 16/e, pp. 1940–1947. McMillan, 3/e, pp. 770–771, 2255. Rudolph, 20/e, pp. 421, 1806–1808.)* The recognition of hearing impairment in a neonate is difficult. The delay in diagnosis that often occurs can seriously jeopardize normal speech development and learning. To aid in early diagnosis, the behavioral or electrophysiologic responses (or both) of infants who are at higher-than-average risk of hearing impairment are monitored closely during the early months of life. Neonatal factors that confer high risk include craniofacial defects (including abnormal ear structure), neonatal asphyxia, bacterial meningitis, congenital infections, significant hyperbilirubinemia, use of ototoxic medications for greater than 5 days, mechanical ventilation for greater than 10 days, stigmata of syndromes causing hearing loss, birth weight less than 1500 g, and family history of deafness. A pattern of malformation that can include hypoplasia of digits, nails, and midface; growth retardation; cardiac defects; and mental deficiency is associated with the maternal use of phenytoin during pregnancy. Hearing loss is not a manifestation of the fetal hydantoin syndrome. The American Academy of Pediatrics has recently recommended universal screening for hearing loss for all newborn infants.

31–32. The answers are 31–c, 32–b. *(Behrman, 16/e, pp. 215–216. McMillan, 3/e, pp. 68–72. Rudolph , 20/e, pp. 1325–1326.)* Rapid expansion of the vascular space is needed. Appropriate intravenous fluids include Ringer's lactate and normal saline. Albumin, plasma, and blood offer no significant advantages over the cheaper and more available Ringer's lactate or normal saline.

In this patient in shock, it is vital to restore blood volume quickly, thereby improving tissue perfusion and shifting anaerobic toward aerobic metabolism. The restoration of vascular volume would also improve functioning of the intestines so that diarrhea will abate and would improve circulation to the kidney so that renal function would be restored. A volume of 20 mL/kg is about one-quarter the blood volume of the patient; therefore it should be given at a rate that will not produce pulmonary edema. An emergency phase lasting 1 to 2 hours or less has worked well in practice.

The dextrose fluids listed are various forms of maintenance fluids.

33. The answer is d. *(Behrman, 16/e, pp. 1348–1349. McMillan, 3/e, pp. 547–548. Rudolph, 20/e, p. 2167.)* Average blood pressure tends to increase with age. Thus, a value of 120/80 mm Hg, clearly acceptable for most adults and children older than about 10 years of age, is in the hypertensive range for much of childhood. In the newborn period, a systolic pressure above 87 mm Hg is considered hypertensive.

34. The answer is a. *(Behrman, 16/e, pp. 777, 779–780. McMillan, 3/e, pp. 416–418. Rudolph, 20/e, p. 578.)* Examination of the joint fluid is the key to diagnosis. The joint tap will reveal cloudy fluid containing a predominance of polymorphonuclear leukocytes. Organisms are readily seen on Gram stain examination; culture of joint fluid and blood are usually positive. X-ray reveals a widened joint space. Finding pus in the joint indicates the need for immediate surgical drainage and prompt institution of IV antibiotic therapy to avoid serious damage to the joint and permanent loss of function. The most common organism found to cause septic arthritis is *Staphylococcus aureus*. Since immunization against *Haemophilus influenzae* type b has become an established practice, invasive disease such as septic arthritis caused by this organism is rarely seen. In sexually active adolescents, *Neisseria gonorrhoeae* is a common cause of septic arthritis.

35. The answer is b. (*Behrman, 16/e, pp. 878–880. McMillan, 3/e, pp. 486–487, 940 Rudolph, 20/e, pp. 612–614.*) The patient should receive a booster immunization with adult Td, which should be given every 10 years to maintain immunity against both diphtheria and tetanus. He does not need passive immunization with tetanus immune globulin because the wound is superficial and there appears to be little or no risk of tetanus. As of 1993, pertussis immunization is discontinued at age 7 years.

36. The answer is a. (*Behrman, 16/e, pp. 790–792. McMillan, 3/e, p. 587.*) Mammalian bites should be promptly and thoroughly scrubbed with soap and water and debrided. The decision to suture depends on the location, age, and nature of the wound. Antibiotic prophylaxis should be considered in cat, human, or monkey bites. Only 4 percent of dog bites become infected (and do not necessarily need antibiotic prophylaxis) compared with 35 percent of cat bites and 50 percent of monkey bites (which require antibiotics in most cases). Cat bites are usually deep punctures. Human bites almost invariably become infected. The etiologies of these infections are polymicrobial. *Pasteurella multocida* is a common organism in infected cat and dog bites. Infected human bites tend to have positive cultures for *Streptococcus viridans, Staphylococcus aureus*, and *Bacteroides* species. Treatment with oral amoxicillin-clavulanate, erythromycin, or, in older children, minocycline is recommended. Antibiotic prophylaxis is recommended for any bite sustained by an infant, a diabetic, or an immunocompromised patient because of the higher risk of infection in these persons.

37. The answer is b. (*Behrman, 16/e, p. 91. McMillan, 3/e, p. 622. Rudolph, 20/e, pp. 851–853.*) Poisoning with tricyclic antidepressants is a leading reason for admissions to pediatric intensive care units and the leading cause of fatal drug overdose in adolescents. These preparations produce a variety of pharmacologic effects, including inhibition of muscarinic/cholinergic receptors, blockade of norepinephrine and serotonin uptake, and depression of sodium channels responsible for cardiac cell membrane depolarization. The toxic-to-therapeutic ratio is low. Young children often ingest poisons and drugs during times of household disruption. Visitors' handbags are a great temptation for the inquisitive toddler.

38. The answer is d. *(Behrman, 16/e, pp. 2156–2159. McMillan, 3/e, pp. 632–633. Rudolph, 20/e, pp. 16–17.)* Because of recent evidence that impairment of cognitive function can occur at blood lead levels previously thought to be safe, the toxic concentration of lead in whole blood was revised downward in 1991 from 25 µg/dL to 10 µg/dL. The blood erythrocyte protoporphyrin concentration is not elevated in low-level poisoning; therefore, testing for erythrocyte protoporphyrin is no longer a valid screen. The definitive screen is the blood lead level. Venipuncture avoids the risk of environmental contamination with lead that is more likely with finger sticks. Most lead poisoning is clinically inapparent. A careful history will help to identify sources of lead in the environment. Neither the history nor the anemia that accompanies severe lead poisoning, however, is an appropriate means of screening for lead poisoning. Some authorities state that screening of the environment and removal of sources of lead is preferable to screening of children.

39. The answer is d. *(Behrman, 16/e, pp. 771–773, 1083–1084. McMillan, 3/e, pp. 447–448, 1724–1725. Rudolph, 20/e, pp. 647–651, 1151.)* In the United States, the hepatitis B virus is transmitted mainly by exposure to blood and blood products, through sexual contact, and from mothers to newborns. Close family contact has also been implicated as a factor in transmission. About one third of cases have no identifiable risk factor. Although the infection usually presents as viral hepatitis, its full impact may not be realized until years later. Chronic active hepatitis is a complication characterized by unresolving inflammation, which can eventually lead to necrosis and fibrosis of the liver and possible progression to cirrhosis and liver failure. Hepatocellular carcinoma is another long-term complication of hepatitis B infection. Acute fulminant hepatitis causes massive destruction of hepatic parenchyma, but is fortunately a rare complication of infection with the virus. Hydrops of the gallbladder is not related to hepatitis B infection. It is usually idiopathic but can be a complication of Kawasaki disease among other diseases.

40. The answer is a. *(Behrman, 16/e, pp. 2139–2143. McMillan, 3/e, p. 602. Rudolph, 20/e, p. 872.)* An increasing number of studies in infants are pointing to the prone (face down) sleeping position as a risk factor for sudden infant death syndrome (SIDS). A higher risk of SIDS in the prone position has been noted when the infant sleeps on a soft, porous mattress or in an overheated room, is swaddled, or has recently been ill. The American Academy of Pediatrics recommends that healthy infants be positioned on their side or back when being put down for sleep. (The prone position is still recommended for infants with certain medical conditions.) The rate of SIDS has declined in areas where the change from prone to supine (face up) sleeping positions has been effected.

41. The answer is d. *(Behrman, 16/e, p. 331. McMillan, 3/e, p. 2232. Rudolph, 20/e, pp. 426–427.)* The physical features associated with the fragile X syndrome become more obvious after puberty. They include a long face, large ears, prominent jaw, macroorchidism, hypotonia, repetitive speech, gaze avoidance, and hand flapping. Even in the absence of physical findings, boys of all ages with developmental delay, autism, and abnormal temperament of unknown cause probably should be tested for the fragile X syndrome.

The genetics of the fragile X syndrome are unique. Most males who carry the fragile X mutation are mentally impaired and show the clinical phenotype; however, 20 percent of males who inherit the genetic mutation are normal in intelligence and physical appearance. They are also cytogenetically normal in that the fragile site on their X chromosome is not seen by the karyotyping method. These normal transmitting males (NTMs) transmit the fragile X mental retardation (FMR-1) gene to all of their daughters and often have severely affected grandchildren. It is thought that a premutation carried by these NTMs must go through oogenesis in their daughters to become a full mutation. Daughters of NTMs are usually normal but are obligate carriers of the FMR-1 gene. Daughters who inherit the gene from the mother are retarded about one third of the time. Because both males and females can be affected, the fragile X syndrome is best described as a dominant X-linked disorder with reduced penetrance in females. Cytogenetic testing for the fragile site on the X chromosome is an unsatisfactory method of identifying persons with this mutation for the following reasons: (1) not all cells in the affected males show the fragile site; (2) NTMs have no fragile X site demonstrable by this method; and (3) a significant percentage of carrier females are cytogenetically normal. In 1991, the FMR-1 gene was cloned. Direct DNA analysis is now available for diagnosis of phenotypically affected persons as well as suspected carriers of fragile X; it can also be used for prenatal testing.

42. The answer is a. (*Behrman, 16/e, pp. 215–216. McMillan, 3/e, p. 68. Rudolph, 20/e, pp. 1325–1326.*) "Normal" saline has an NaCl concentration of 0.9 percent (9 g/L or 154 mEq/L). This makes it isotonic with blood and body fluids so that it will not cause osmotic hemolysis or damage to tissues or vascular channels. The ratio of Na+ to Cl- is not physiologic because that ratio in blood is 140 to 100. Lactate and glucose are not included in plain normal saline.

43–48. The answers are 43–e, 44–b, 45–d, 46–a, 47–g, 48–f. (*Behrman, 16/e, pp. 1971–1972, 1983, 1996–1997. McMillan, 3/e, pp. 373, 375–377, 380, 683–684, 690, 706, 723, 730. Rudolph pp. 211–212, 883–884, 887.*) Erythema toxicum is a benign, self-limited condition of unknown etiology. It is found in about 50 percent of term newborns. Lesions are yellow-white and 1- to 2-mm in size with a surrounding edge of erythema. This rash waxes and wanes over the first days to weeks of life. Examination of the fluid from these lesions demonstrates eosinophils. No therapy is indicated.

Salmon patches are flat vascular lesions that occur in the listed regions and appear more prominent during crying. The lesions on the face fade over the first weeks of life. Lesions found over the nuchal and occipital areas often persist. No therapy is indicated.

Pustular melanosis is another benign, self-limited disease of unknown etiology found during the newborn period. It is more common in blacks than in whites. These lesions are usually found at birth and consist of 1- to 2-mm pustules that result in a hyperpigmented lesion upon rupture of the pustule. The pustular stage of these lesions occurs during the first few days of life with the hyperpigmented stage lasting for weeks to months. No therapy is indicated.

Sebaceous nevi (nevus of Jadassohn) are small, sharply edged lesions that occur most commonly on the head and neck of infants. These lesions are yellow-orange in color and are slightly elevated. They usually are hairless. Malignant degeneration is possible, most commonly after adolescence.

Milia are fine, yellowish white, 1- to 2-mm lesions scattered over the face and gingivae of the neonate. They are cysts that contain keratinized material. Commonly, these lesions resolve spontaneously without therapy.

Seborrheic dermatitis can begin anytime during life and frequently presents as cradle cap in the newborn period. This rash is commonly greasy, scaly, and erythematous and in smaller children involves the face, neck, axilla, and diaper area. In older children, the rash can be localized to the scalp and intertriginous areas. Pruritus can be marked.

49–53. The answers are 49–c, 50–c, 51–b, 52–e, 53–e. _(Behrman, 16/e, pp. 817–820, 833–837, 878–880, 946–953. McMillan, 3/e, pp. 479–491. Rudolph, 20/e, pp. 30–36.)_ The diphtheria bacillus causes a disease characterized by the formation of a pseudomembrane in the upper respiratory tract, which can obstruct the airway, and by the elaboration of an exotoxin that interferes with cellular protein synthesis and causes widespread damage to visceral organs and the CNS. The use of diphtheria toxoid combined with tetanus toxoid and pertussis vaccine (DTP) according to the recommended schedule will maintain a protective level of antitoxin against diphtheria.

The manifestations of tetanus are due to an exotoxin elaborated by the vegetative form of _Clostridium tetani._ Active immunization of all children with tetanus toxoid according to the recommended schedule and continued administration of boosters every 10 years will maintain a protective level of antitoxin throughout a person's lifetime.

The outermost structure of the gram-negative organism _Haemophilus influenzae_ is its polysaccharide capsule. Of the six distinct polysaccharide types, type b is the most significant clinically because it accounts for most invasive disease, such as meningitis, epiglottitis, septic arthritis, and cellulitis. Vaccines have been designed to induce antibodies against poly-ribose ribitol phosphate (PRP), the capsular polysaccharide of _H. influenzae_ type b. Conjugation of the antigen to a protein has enhanced its immunogenicity such that it acts as a T-cell-dependent antigen, developing immunologic memory and thereby inducing an anamnestic response on reexposure to the antigen.

A number of vaccines against measles have been developed since the isolation of the virus in tissue culture in 1954. The administration of the attenuated live viral vaccines currently in use produces specific antibodies by causing an infection that is mild or asymptomatic, noncommunicable, and unassociated with secondary bacterial infection or neurologic complications.

Seroconversion results from immunization with live attenuated rubella viral vaccine in almost all susceptible persons. A mild or asymptomatic infection occurs, which results in active antibody production. Apparently, spread of vaccine virus from vaccinated to susceptible persons does not occur.

54–58. The answers are 54–b, 55–c, 56–d, 57–a, 58–c. (Behrman, 16/e, pp. 231–237. McMillan, 3/e, pp. 497, 499–502. Rudolph, pp. 20–21, 27–29, 857.) The majority of deaths due to asphyxia or choking are due to food items (hot dogs, candy, grapes, and occasionally to nonfood items such as pacifiers, balloons, and small toys).

Drowning risks are age-dependent. Most drownings are accidental. Infants drown in bathtubs; unsupervised toddlers and young children fall into swimming pools, ponds, and streams. Alcohol and drugs are factors in many teenage drownings. Swimming pool drownings generally occur between ages 1 and 3 years. It is essential to counsel parents never to allow young children to swim or bathe unsupervised. Pools should be fenced and meticulous attention must be paid to locking the gate.

Pedestrian injuries are the leading cause of death due to trauma in 5- to 9-year-old children and are most likely to occur in boys. Parents should be advised to dress children who play outdoors in brightly colored, reflective clothing and to teach them the fundamentals of pedestrian safety.

Baby walkers are popular with many parents who believe erroneously that they are helpful to a baby who is learning to walk. They increase mobilization of an infant, which increases the infant's risks to those of a more mobile toddler.

The Poison Prevention Packaging Act of 1970 achieved considerable success in reducing the number of accidental poisonings in children by mandating the manufacture of child-resistant containers, reducing the quantity of drug in a container to safer limits, and ordering the printing of warnings on container labels. Despite of these safeguards, children are still at risk of accidental poisonings, especially children less than 5 years of age. These accidents are more likely to occur when children are left unattended or unsupervised and when there is a disruption in the usual family routines. Anticipatory guidance regarding accidental ingestion is an essential part of well-child medical care.

59–62. The answers are 59–a, 60–c, 61–b, 62–d. *(Behrman, 16/e, pp. 169, 179–181, 184–187, 2054. McMillan, 3/e, 470–475. Rudolph, pp. 1007–1010, 1015.)* Marasmus (infantile atrophy) is due to inadequate caloric intake that can be linked with such factors as insufficient food resources, poor feeding techniques, metabolic disorders, and congenital anomalies. Patients with marasmus have progressive weight loss, constipation, muscular atrophy, loss of skin turgor, hypothermia, and possibly, edema. In advanced disease, affected infants are lethargic and can have starvation diarrhea, with small, mucus-containing stools. These children appear emaciated and cachetic.

Pellagra, which literally means "rough skin," is due to a deficiency of niacin (nicotinic acid). Niacin is an essential component of two enzymes—nicotinamide adenine dinucleotide (NAD) and nicotinamide adenine dinucleotide phosphate (NADP)—that are needed for electron transfer and glycolysis. Pellagra is most prevalent in areas that rely on corn as a basic foodstuff (corn contains little tryptophan, which can be converted into niacin). The classic (3-D) triad of clinical symptoms of pellagra consists of dermatitis, diarrhea, and dementia, although classic symptoms are not well developed in infants.

Beriberi results from a deficiency of thiamine (vitamin B_1), which is essential for the synthesis of acetylcholine and for the operation of certain enzyme systems in carbohydrate metabolism. Thiamine is present in fair amounts in breast milk, cow's milk, cereals, fruits, vegetables, and eggs; meat and legumes are good sources. Thiamine is destroyed by heat and cooking in water, and polishing of grains reduces their thiamine content by removing the coverings that contain most of the vitamin. Clinical disturbances stemming from thiamine deficiency are congestive heart failure, peripheral neuritis, and psychic disturbances.

Rickets is a disorder of growing bone characterized by defective mineralization of matrix. Rickets that responds to administration of physiologic doses of vitamin D is termed vitamin D-deficient rickets. Deficiency of vitamin D can lead to osseous changes, such as enlargement of the costochondral junctions ("rachitic rosary") and craniotabes, within a few months; advanced rickets can cause scoliosis, pelvic and leg deformities, "pigeon breast," rachitic dwarfism, and other disorders. It is most commonly seen in industrialized nations in black children, children undergoing rapid growth (low-birthweight infants and adolescents), and children with malabsorption syndromes.

63–66. The answers are 63–b, 64–c, 65–d, 66–a. *(Behrman 16/e, pp. 350, 1699, 1903, 1919, 1922, 1984, 1986. McMillan, 3/e, pp. 667, 712, 2251. Rudolph, 20/e, pp. 904, 945–946, 1759, 1802, 2101.)* Waardenburg's syndrome is the most common of several syndromes that are characterized by both deafness and pigmentary changes. Features of this syndrome, which is inherited as an autosomal dominant disorder, include a distinctive white forelock, heterochromia irides, unilateral or bilateral congenital deafness, and lateral displacement of the inner canthi.

People who have Pendred's syndrome, inherited as an autosomal recessive trait, typically have a marked hearing loss and thyroid dysfunction. Goiter, which usually develops before affected children reach the age of 10 years, can arise because their thyroid glands are unable to convert inorganic iodine into organic iodine. The benign goiter responds to thyroid replacement therapy.

Congenital deafness is also a symptom of the autosomal recessive Usher's syndrome. Pigmentary changes in the retina (retinitis pigmentosa) can be detected in affected infants, and these degenerative changes continue throughout life. Early visual impairments include loss of night vision and development of tunnel vision. Functional blindness can arise in affected adolescents and adults.

LEOPARD syndrome is characterized by the presence of multiple **L**entigines, **E**lectrocardiographic changes, **O**cular hypertelorism, **P**ulmonary stenosis, **A**bnormal genitalia, **R**etardation of growth, and profound **D**eafness. The syndrome is inherited as an autosomal dominant disorder with variable penetrance.

67–70. The answers are 67–a, 68–b, 69–d, 70–e. *(Behrman, 16/e, pp. 2080–2084, 2092. McMillan, 3/e, 2105–2106, 2117, 2123. Rudolph, 20/e, pp. 2145–2148, 2153–2155.)* Legg-Calvé-Perthes disease is avascular necrosis or idiopathic osteonecrosis of the femoral head; the cause of this disorder is unknown. Boys between the ages of 2 and 12 years are most frequently affected (incidence in boys greater by four- to fivefold; mean of 6 to 7 years old). Presenting symptoms include a limp and pain in the anterior thigh, groin, or knee, although classic symptoms include a painless limp.

Slipped capital femoral epiphysis is a disease of unknown etiology and occurs typically in adolescents; the disorder is most common among obese boys with delayed skeletal maturation or in thin, tall adolescents having recently enjoyed a growth spurt. Onset of this disorder is frequently gradual; pain referred to the knee in 20 percent of cases can mask the hip pathology.

Idiopathic scoliosis occurs slightly more frequently in adolescent girls than boys, but progresses to require treatment far more commonly in girls than boys. This condition requires prompt evaluation. Treatment by bracing, spinal fusion, or both is sometimes necessary. As many as 70 percent of children with scoliosis have family members with this disease.

Subluxation of the head of the radius occurs most commonly in children who are 1 to 4 years of age and have been jerked forcibly by the hand. Affected children have pain in the elbow and are unable to supinate the forearm. The diagnosis is established if supination of the forearm, while the elbow is stabilized, corrects the subluxation.

71–75. The answers are 71–c, 72–b, 73–d, 74–e, 75 a. (*Behrman, 16/e, pp. 2160–2167. McMillan, 3/e, pp. 620–621, 623–627, 629–635. Rudolph, 20/e, pp. 813, 817 818, 835–837, 841–843, 847–849.*) The most important aspect of the management of lead poisoning is the identification and withdrawal of the source of the lead. Patients with symptomatic lead poisoning or high lead levels in the blood (over 70 μg/dL) should be treated with both dimercaprol and calcium EDTA. With milder poisoning, intravenous or intramuscular calcium EDTA or more likely oral dimercaptosuccinic acid can be used.

N-acetylcysteine (NAC) is effective treatment of acetaminophen poisoning and acts by removing hepatotoxic metabolites. It should be given within 16 h of ingestion; after 36 h it is probably ineffective.

Morphine and other narcotics produce their major toxic effect by suppression of ventilation. Ventilatory support can be necessary initially, but naloxone is a specific antidote and can be very rapidly effective. The effect of naloxone can wear off more quickly than the effects of the drug for which it was given, so careful observation and repeated doses may be necessary.

Salicylate poisoning is not treated with any of these drugs. It produces metabolic acidosis and respiratory alkalosis (although this latter feature is often missed in young children), hyperglycemia and hypoglycemia, dehydration, and lethargy. Excretion of salicylates in the urine can be markedly enhanced by the administration of acetazolamide and intravenous sodium bicarbonate. Hemodialysis can also be used.

Organophosphate insecticides are absorbed from all sites and act by inhibiting cholinesterases, thereby leading to the accumulation of high levels of acetylcholine. This affects the parasympathetic nervous system, muscle, and the central nervous system. Treatment of a patient contaminated with organophosphate insecticide will include thorough washing of the pesticide from the skin, inducing emesis or performing gastric lavage, supporting ventilation, and administering atropine followed by pralidoxime (2-PAM).

76–78. The answers are 76–b, 77–a, 78–d. (Behrman, 16/e, pp. 2160–2169. McMillan, 3/e, pp. 620–621. Rudolph, 20/e, pp. 831–832, 851–852.) Phenothiazine toxicity can cause extrapyramidal symptoms such as oculogyric crisis, tremors, and dysphagia. These dystonic symptoms respond surprisingly quickly to the intravenous or intramuscular administration of diphenhydramine (Benadryl).

Iron in the form of salts such as ferrous sulfate or gluconate used to treat iron deficiency anemia can be highly toxic to infants; as few as three tablets can cause severe symptoms and as few as 10 tablets can be lethal to young children. Symptoms occur in two phases: gastrointestinal symptoms such as bloody vomiting or diarrhea and abdominal pain, followed by a latent period of up to 12 h or more and terminating with cardiovascular collapse. Deferoxamine given intravenously or intramuscularly forms a complex with the iron and is excreted in the urine, to which it imparts the color of vin rosé (red wine).

Methanol, also known as methyl alcohol or wood alcohol, is present in a number of household products. Toxicity causes a profound metabolic acidosis. Treatment includes emptying the stomach by inducing emesis or by gastric lavage, the intravenous infusion of ethanol to saturate the enzyme systems that convert methanol to toxins, and in severe poisoning, the use of hemodialysis to remove the methanol.

79–83. The answers are 79–d, 80–g, 81–a, 82–e, 83–b. (Behrman, 16/e, pp. 146–147, 178, 181–184, 187–188. McMillan, 3/e, pp. 83–84, 474–475, 1752. Rudolph, pp. 1007–1009.) So far, there is very little or no well-documented clinical evidence to justify the use of large doses of vitamins beyond the levels found in a regular, balanced diet. Vitamin excess can be dangerous. Vitamin A in large doses slows growth and causes hyperostosis (excess bone growth), hepatomegaly, increased CSF pressure, and drying of skin. Nicotinic acid, a vasodilator, causes skin flushing and pruritus; long-term use can cause tachycardia, liver damage, hyperglycemia, and hyperuricemia. Excessive doses of vitamin C, in addition to causing kidney stones, diarrhea, and cramps, increase the normal requirement for the vitamin when large doses are discontinued. Prolonged excessive intake of vitamin D can cause nausea, diarrhea, weight loss, polyuria, and soft-tissue calcification of heart, kidney, blood vessels, bronchi, and stomach. Excessive intake of pyridoxine (B_6) can result in sensory neuropathy with altered sensation of touch, pain, and fever.

84–88. The answers are 84–f, 85–b, 86–d, 87–a, 88–e. (*Behrman, 16/e, pp. 468–469, 473, 716. McMillan, 3/e, pp. 2165, 2227–2228, Rudolph, 20/e, pp. 419–421, 909.*) The fetal environment is affected by factors that alter maternal metabolism, among them diseases such as juvenile-onset insulin-dependent diabetes mellitus and lupus erythematosus. Infants of diabetic mothers have a two to three times greater risk than the general population of having anomalies. These anomalies include sacral agenesis (which is pathognomonic for maternal diabetes mellitus), cardiac defects (e.g., transposition of the great arteries and ventricular septal defects), renal defects, and anencephaly.

The use of the anticonvulsants phenytoin and valproate during pregnancy to control seizures has been associated with findings of fetal malformation. Prenatal exposure to phenytoin can result in the characteristic features of the fetal hydantoin syndrome: pre- and postnatal growth retardation, hypoplasia of distal phalanges and nails, and alterations in central nervous system performance. The incidence of neural tube defects in the fetus can be increased in mothers receiving valproate during the first trimester of pregnancy. Although the risk (1 percent to 2 percent, as estimated by the Centers for Disease Control) is similar to that for nonepileptic women who have had children with neural tube defects, caution is advised in the use of this drug during pregnancy.

Heavy alcohol ingestion is associated with a syndrome (fetal alcohol syndrome) consisting of pre- and postnatal growth retardation, developmental delay, and a characteristic facies that includes microcephaly, microphthalmia, and a flattened philtrum area. Skeletal, joint, and cardiac abnormalities have also been associated with this syndrome. It has been stated that infants of mothers who drink heavily (>3 oz of absolute alcohol daily) have a 30 percent to 50 percent risk of abnormalities of growth and performance. No safe amount of alcohol consumption during pregnancy is known; therefore, pregnant women and those who might become pregnant should be advised to abstain from alcohol.

The clinical findings associated with neonatal lupus erythematosus include skin lesions and cardiac abnormalities, among them AV block (which is a permanent condition), complete transposition of the great arteries, and valvular and septal defects. Most mothers are symptomatic prior to or during pregnancy, but occasionally the diagnosis of lupus in the mother is made when her newborn is found to have heart block. Most babies with lupus erythematosus will have anti-Ro antibodies, which are considered markers for the disease. Antinuclear antibodies, which are also present in most infants, also disappear by 6 months of age.

89–92. The answers are 89–b, 90–e, 91–d, 92–a. *(Behrman, 16/e, pp. 680–684, 2028–2029, 2042–2046, McMillan, 3/e, pp. 688–689, 702, 704–706, 716–717, 2059–2063. Rudolph, 20/e, pp. 469–473, 780–781, 889–892, 929, 935–936, 938.)* Impetigo is a common skin condition of children that begins on the face or extremities after the skin has been traumatized. The two organisms that cause most of the infections are *Staphylococcus aureus* and ß-hemolytic streptococci. In most cases, a tiny vesicle or pustule forms, which rapidly degenerates into a honey-colored, crusty plaque. Usually no pain or systemic symptoms are associated with these lesions. Complications are rare, but acute post-streptococcal glomerulonephritis is possible. Treatment is by topical or systemic antibiotics.

Scabies is caused by mites (*Sarcoptes scabiei* var. *hominis*), which burrow into the skin and release toxins that result in extremely pruritic lesions. These lesions range from a threadlike burrow in older patients to bullae and pustules in infants. Common sites of infection in older patients are the interdigital spaces, wrist, axillary folds, ankles, buttocks, and groin. An infant's most common locations are feet, palms, axilla, and scalp. The lesions are rarely found above the neck in older children. The diagnosis can be made either clinically or by microscopic identification of the mites. Therapy consists of treatment with either 1% lindane (not in smaller children) or permethrin 5% cream (less toxicity for smaller children).

Molluscum contagiosum is caused by a poxvirus. Lesions are skin-colored, dome-shaped, and about 1 to 5 mm in size. They can be distinguished by the central umbilication found on most lesions. Areas of predilection include the face, eyelids, neck, axillae, and thighs. Diagnosis can usually be made on clinical grounds. Therapy includes observation (the disease can be self-limited), application of liquid nitrogen to the lesion, extrusion of the central plug with a needle or curette, or a topical application of cantharidin 0.9% to each lesion.

Atopic dermatitis, an immediate hypersensitivity reaction to common environmental irritants, has a prevalence of 2 percent to 3 percent in children. Inflammatory patches and weeping, crusted plaques on the neck, face, groin, and extensor surfaces characterize the infantile form. In older children, dermatitis of the flexural areas is common. Soaps and hot water are common irritants. Therapy is based on avoidance of irritants, adequate hydration of the skin, and use of topical steroids, as well as treatment of infected lesions.

93–95. The answers are 93–d, 94–a, 95–c. (*Behrman, 16/e, pp. 716, 1369–1371, 1575–1576, 1581–1582. McMillan, 3/e, pp. 381, 1354–1357, 1581–1598, 2165. Rudolph, 20/e, pp. 909, 1351–1358, 1466–1468.*) The ventricular septal defect is the most common congenital cardiac malformation. Although small lesions result in insignificant left-to-right shunts, the murmur associated with them can be significantly louder due to turbulent blood flow. Larger lesions result in significant left-to-right shunting of blood and can result in dyspnea, poor growth, and heart failure, usually during early infancy.

The classic presentation of acute poststreptococcal glomerulonephritis consists of the sudden onset of change in urine color (bloody), edema, hypertension, and renal insufficiency. This disease follows an infection of the throat or the skin with a nephrogenic strain of group A ß-hemolytic streptococci. The oliguria can progress to heart failure if fluid overload occurs.

Neonatal lupus can be responsible for a variety of problems in the newborn. Mothers with antibodies to Ro/SSA and some with antibodies to La/SSB can deliver infants with rashes, thrombocytopenia, and congenital heart block among the more common problems. Whereas the other symptoms usually resolve during the first months of life, the congenital heart block can be irreversible and can result in heart failure, need for early pacemakers, and an increased incidence of early death.

96–102. The answers are 96–b, 97–f, 98–c, 99–a, 100–d, 101–f, 102–e. (*Behrman, 16/e, pp. 151, 178, 459, 1163–1164, 1467–1468, 1474. McMillan, 3/e, 367, 477, 1035–1036, 1487–1488, 1753–1754. Rudolph, 20/e, pp. 23, 227, 234, 621, 665, 1162–1163, 1181–1182, 1205–1206, 2188.*) Isoniazid therapy can cause peripheral neuritis as a result of competitive inhibition of pyridoxine metabolism when the dose is high and the patient is poorly nourished or alcoholic. It is seldom seen in childhood. To be safe, vitamin B_6 supplements should be given to adolescents. Children maintained on anticonvulsants can develop low folate levels that, rarely, can be associated with megaloblastic anemia. Folic acid supplementation may be indicated.

The WHO recommends that in communities where vitamin A deficiency is prevalent, vitamin A should be given to all children with measles. Compliance with this recommendation has resulted in a definite reduction in measles-related morbidity and mortality. In the United States, vitamin A supplements should be considered for use in measles patients with immunodeficiency, impaired intestinal absorption, and malnutrition. Recent immigrants from areas with a high mortality from measles and who show ophthalmologic evidence of vitamin A deficiency (blindness, Bitot's spots, or xerophthalmia), should also be included in that group.

Fat malabsorption occurs (1) in the absence of pancreatic enzymes, as in cystic fibrosis; (2) as a result of failure of micellar solubilization by bile salts, as in chronic liver disease; and (3) with a problematic mucosal uptake, as in celiac sprue. In these conditions, attention must be paid to the provision of fat-soluble vitamins A, D, E, and K.

Both human and cow's milk are low in vitamin D content. Cow's milk and infant formulas are fortified with this vitamin. Breast-fed infants require supplementation with vitamin D, particularly when adequate exposure to sunlight cannot be assured, such as in urban areas where pollutants obscure ultraviolet light, and in patients with darkly pigmented skin.

Patients with hemolytic anemia, such as sickle cell disease, have an ongoing compensatory erythropoiesis. To supply the increased need of rapidly dividing red blood cell precursors for folate, supplementation is necessary.

In newborns, a lack of free vitamin K in the mother and the absence of bacterial intestinal flora that synthesizes vitamin K result in a transient deficiency in vitamin K-dependent factors (II, VI, IX, X). Milk is a poor source of vitamin K. Vitamin K administered shortly after birth prevents hemorrhagic disease of the newborn.

103–107. The answers are 103–c, 104–f, 105–b, 106–g, 107–e. (*Behrman, 16/e, p. 617. McMillan, 3/e, pp. 2091–2092. Rudolph, 20/e, pp. 437–439.*)The bulk of immunodeficiencies can be ruled out with little cost. Wiskott-Aldrich syndrome is unlikely if the platelet count is normal.

Asplenia results in Howell-Jolly bodies, so a complete blood count can rule out this disease. B-cell defects are likely to result in low immunoglobulin A, G, and M levels. An intradermal skin test using *Candida albicans* will result in no response in the patient with T-cell deficiencies. The nitroblue tetrazolium or other respiratory burst assay will help identify phagocytic-cell defects such as chronic granulomatous disease. Should any of these tests prove to be positive, more extensive, invasive, and expensive testing can be undertaken.

THE NEWBORN INFANT

Questions

DIRECTIONS: Each item below contains a question or incomplete statement followed by suggested responses. Select the **one best** response to each question.

108. The infant pictured as follows was small for gestational age. He also was found to have a ventricular septal defect on cardiac evaluation. This infant appeared to have features consistent with

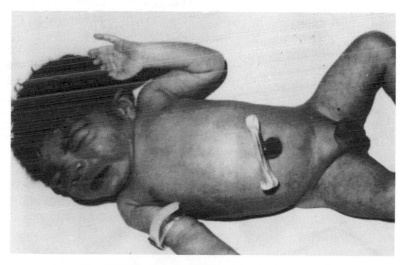

(From Karp RJ (ed). *Malnourished Children in the United States.*
New York: Springer Publishing; 1993, with permission.)

a. perinatal phenytoin exposure
b. trisomy 21
c. Alport's syndrome
d. fetal alcohol syndrome
e. infant of diabetic mother

109. A newborn is noted to be quite jaundiced at 3 days of age. Which of the following factors is associated with an increased risk of neurologic damage in a jaundice newborn?

a. metabolic alkalosis
b. increased attachment of bilirubin to binding sites caused by drugs such as sulfisoxazole
c. hyperalbuminemia
d. neonatal sepsis
e. maternal ingestion of phenobarbital during pregnancy

110. A full-term newborn infant is having episodes of cyanosis and apnea, which are worse when he is attempting to feed, but he seems better when he is crying. The most important next step to establish quickly the diagnosis is

a. echocardiogram
b. ventilation perfusion scan
c. passage of catheter into nose
d. hemoglobin electrophoresis
e. bronchoscopic evaluation of palate and larynx

111. The mother of a 7-day-old infant has developed chickenpox. Which of the following is the most appropriate measure?

a. isolate the infant from the mother
b. hospitalize the infant in the isolation ward
c. administer acyclovir to the infant
d. administer varicella-zoster immunoglobulin to the infant
e. advise the mother to continue regular well-baby care for the infant

112. A 2-week-old infant has had no immunizations, sleeps 18 h a day, weighs 3.5 kg, and takes 60 mL of standard infant formula four times a day, but no solid food and no iron or vitamin supplements. Of most concern is

a. immunization status
b. caloric intake
c. iron levels
d. levels of vitamins A, C, and D
e. circadian rhythm

113. A mother delivers a neonate with meconium staining and Apgar scores of 3 at 1 and 5 min of life. She had no prenatal care and the delivery was by emergency cesarean section for severe fetal bradycardia. Which of the following sequelae could be expected to develop in this intubated neonate with respiratory distress?

a. sustained rise in systemic blood pressure
b. hyperactive bowel sounds
c. microcephaly
d. cataracts
e. thrombocytosis

114. A 2-year-old boy is being followed for congenital cytomegalovirus (CMV) infection. He is deaf and developmentally delayed. The child's mother informs you that she has just become pregnant and is concerned that the new baby will be infected. Which of the following is true?

a. the mother has antibodies to CMV that are passed to the fetus
b. the mother's infection cannot become reactivated
c. the likelihood that the new baby will become clinically ill is approximately 80 percent
d. termination of pregnancy is advised
e. the new infant should be isolated from the older child

115. A full-term infant is born after a normal pregnancy; delivery, however, is complicated by marginal placental separation. At 12 h of age the child, although appearing to be in good health, passes a bloody meconium stool. For determining the cause of the bleeding, which of the following diagnostic procedures should be performed first?

a. a barium enema
b. an Apt test
c. gastric lavage with normal saline
d. an upper gastrointestinal series
e. a platelet count, prothrombin time, and partial thromboplastin time

116. Which of the following patterns noted on continuous monitoring of fetal heart rate is most indicative of fetal distress?

a. baseline variability with periodic acceleration
b. increasing baseline variability (saltatory pattern)
c. early deceleration pattern
d. late deceleration without baseline variability
e. variable deceleration with baseline variability

117. Which of the following agents is commonly associated with congenital infections?

a. *Toxoplasma gondii*
b. Group A ß hemolytic streptococcus
c. *Mycobacterium tuberculosis*
d. *Trichomonas*
e. Rotavirus

118. A recovering premature infant who weighs 950 g (2 lb, 1 oz) is fed breast milk to provide 120 cal/kg per day. Over ensuing weeks, the baby is most apt to develop

a. hypernatremia
b. hypocalcemia
c. blood in the stool
d. hyperphosphatemia
e. vitamin D toxicity

119. An infant weighing 1400 g (3 lb) is born at 32 weeks' gestation in a delivery room that has an ambient temperature of 24°C (75°F). If left in an open crib for a few minutes, this child is likely to demonstrate

a. ruddy complexion
b. shivering
c. hypertension
d. increased respiratory rate
e. metabolic alkalosis

120. A primiparous woman whose blood type is O positive gives birth at term to an infant who has A-positive blood and a hematocrit of 55 percent. A serum bilirubin level obtained at 36 h of age is 12 mg/dL. Which of the following laboratory findings would be LEAST characteristic of ABO hemolytic disease?

a. an elevated reticulocyte count
b. a negative direct Coombs' test
c. fragmented red blood cells in the blood smear
d. nucleated red blood cells in the blood smear
e. spherocytes on blood smear

121. Two infants are born at 36 weeks' gestation. Infant A weighs 2600 g (5 lb, 12 oz) and infant B weighs 1600 g (3 lb, 8 oz). Infant B is more likely to have which of the following problems?

a. congenital malformations
b. low hematocrit
c. hyperglycemia
d. surfactant deficiency
e. rapid catch up growth retardation

122. A 3-day-old infant born at 32 weeks' gestation and weighing 1700 g (3 lb, 12 oz) has three episodes of apnea, each lasting 20 to 25 sec and occurring after a feeding. During these episodes, the heart rate drops from 140 to 100 beats per min and the child remains motionless; between episodes, however, the child displays normal activity. Blood sugar is 50 mg/dL and serum calcium is normal. The child's apneic periods most likely are

a. due to an immature respiratory center
b. a part of periodic breathing
c. secondary to hypoglycemia
d. manifestations of seizures
e. evidence of underlying pulmonary disease

Items 123–124

123. You are seeing a 2-week-old boy at a routine visit. The mother complains that he has been constipated, jaundiced, sluggish, and excessively sleepy. The physical examination is normal except for mild jaundice and a distended abdomen in a sleepy infant. Since you suspect hypothyroidism, the most appropriate course to pursue initially is assessment of

a. the mother's serum for auto-antibodies
b. the mother's thyroid status
c. the results of the neonatal metabolic screen
d. levels of thyrotropin-releasing hormone (TRH), thyroid-stimulating hormone (TSH), tri-iodothyronine (T_3), reverse T_3, levothyroxine (T_4), and thyroglobulin in the infant
e. effects on growth and symptoms of a change in feeding practice

124. The most appropriate next step is to

a. obtain a report of repeats of all the abnormal results
b. obtain x-rays of the skull, wrists, and knees
c. start treatment with oral sodium-L-thyroxine, 10 to 15 μg/kg per day
d. evaluate effects of symptomatic treatment for 2 weeks
e. obtain an endocrinology consultation within 2 weeks

Items 125–126

125. A 1-day-old infant who was born by a difficult forceps delivery is alert and active. She does not move her left arm, however, which she keeps internally rotated by her side with the forearm extended and pronated; she also does not move it during a Moro reflex. The rest of her physical examination is normal. This clinical picture most likely indicates

a. fracture of the left clavicle
b. fracture of the left humerus
c. left-sided Erb-Duchenne paralysis
d. left-sided Klumpke's paralysis
e. spinal injury with left hemiparesis

126. The infant in the previous question immediately develops tachypnea with cyanosis. She improves somewhat on oxygen but has predominantly thoracic breathing movements, and the chest x-ray, which appears to have been taken inadvertently at expiration, seems normal. The procedure most likely to provide a specific etiologic diagnosis is

a. venous blood gas
b. CT scan of the head
c. ultrasound or fluoroscopy of the chest
d. bronchoalveolar lavage
e. blood culture

127. A 19-year-old primiparous woman develops toxemia in her last trimester of pregnancy and during the course of her labor is treated with magnesium sulfate. At 38 weeks of gestation, she delivers a 2100-g infant with Apgar scores of 1 and 5 at 1 and 5 minutes, respectively. Laboratory studies at 18 h of age reveal a hematocrit of 79 percent, platelet count of 100,000, glucose 38 mg/dL, magnesium 2.5 mEq/L, and calcium 8.7 mg/dL. Soon after this the infant has a generalized convulsion. The most likely cause of the infant's seizure is

a. polycythemia
b. hypoglycemia
c. hypocalcemia
d. hypermagnesemia
e. thrombocytopenia

128. An infant who appears to be of normal size is noted to be lethargic and somewhat limp after birth. The mother is 28 years old and this is her fourth delivery. The pregnancy was uncomplicated with normal fetal monitoring prior to delivery. Labor was rapid with local anesthesia and intravenous meperidine administered for maternal pain control. Which of the following therapeutic maneuvers is likely to improve this infant's condition most rapidly?

a.   intravenous infusion of 10% dextrose in water
b.   administration of naloxone (Narcan)
c.   administration of vitamin K
d.   measurement of electrolytes and magnesium levels
e.   neurologic consult

129. At 43 weeks' gestation a long, thin infant is delivered who is apneic, limp, pale, and covered with "pea soup" amniotic fluid. The first step in the resuscitation of this infant at delivery should be

a.   suction of the trachea under direct vision
b.   artificial ventilation with bag and mask
c.   artificial ventilation with endotracheal tube
d.   administration of 100% oxygen by mask
e.   catheterization of the umbilical vein

130. A newborn has puffy eyelids, red conjunctivae, and a small amount of clear ocular discharge 6 h after birth. The most likely diagnosis is

a.   dacryocystitis
b.   chemical conjunctivitis
c.   pneumococcal ophthalmia
d.   gonococcal ophthalmia
e.   chlamydial conjunctivitis

131. After an uneventful labor and delivery, an infant is born at 32 weeks' gestation weighing 1500 g (3 lb, 5 oz). Respiratory difficulty develops immediately after birth and increases in intensity thereafter. The child's mother (gravida 3, para 2, no abortions) previously lost an infant because of hyaline membrane disease. At 6 h of age, the child's respiratory rate is 60 breaths per min. Examination reveals grunting, intercostal retraction, nasal flaring, and marked cyanosis in room air. Physiologic abnormalities compatible with these data include

a.   decreased lung compliance, reduced lung volume, left-to-right shunt of blood
b.   decreased lung compliance, reduced lung volume, right-to-left shunt of blood
c.   decreased lung compliance, increased lung volume, left-to-right shunt of blood
d.   normal lung compliance, reduced lung volume, left-to-right shunt of blood
e.   normal lung compliance, increased lung volume, right-to-left shunt of blood

132. Which of the following findings would necessitate further evaluation in a 2000-g newborn infant with appropriate weight for gestation age?

a. positive glabellar tap reflex
b. incomplete scarf sign
c. equivocal plantar response
d. incomplete Moro response
e. serpentine tongue movements

133. Initial examination of a full-term infant weighing less than 2500 g (5 lb, 8 oz) shows edema over the dorsum of her hands and feet. Which of the following findings would support a diagnosis of Turner's syndrome?

a. a liver palpable to 2 cm below the costal margin
b. tremulous movements and ankle clonus
c. redundant skin folds at the nape of the neck
d. a transient, longitudinal division of the body into a red half and a pale half
e. softness of the parietal bones at the vertex

134. A 1-week-old black infant presents to you for the first time with a large, fairly well-defined, purple lesion over the buttocks bilaterally as shown in the photograph. The lesion is not palpable, and it is not warm or tender. The mother denies trauma and reports that the lesion has been present since birth. This otherwise well-appearing infant is growing and developing normally and appears normal upon physical examination. The most likely diagnosis in this infant is

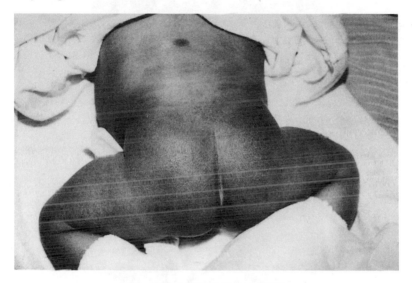

(Courtesy Adelaide Hebert, M.D.)

a. child abuse
b. mongolian spot
c. subcutaneous fat necrosis
d. vitamin K deficiency
e. hemophilia

135. A newborn infant develops respiratory distress immediately after birth. His abdomen is scaphoid. No breath sounds are heard on the left side of his chest, but they are audible on the right. Immediate intubation is successful with little or no improvement in clinical status. Emergency chest x-ray is shown (**A**) along with an x-ray 2 hours later (**B**). The most likely explanation for this infant's condition is

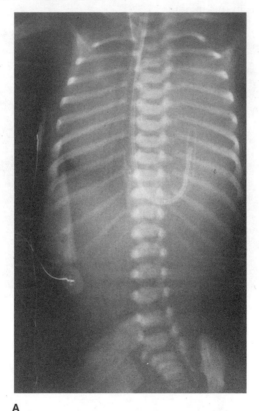

A

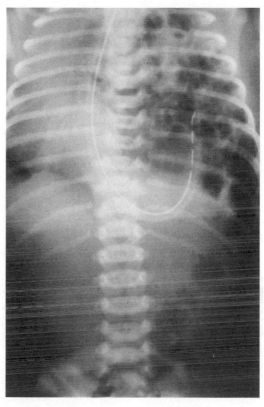

B   (Courtesy Susan John, M.D.)

a. pneumonia
b. cyanotic heart disease
c. diaphragmatic hernia
d. choanal atresia
e. pneumothorax

136. Shortly after birth, an infant develops abdominal distention and begins to drool. When she is given her first feeding, it runs out the side of her mouth and she coughs and chokes. Physical examination reveals tachypnea, intercostal retractions, and bilateral pulmonary rales. The esophageal anomaly that most commonly causes these signs and symptoms is illustrated by

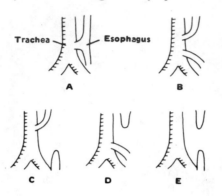

a. figure **A**
b. figure **B**
c. figure **C**
d. figure **D**
e. figure **E**

137. Failure to administer vitamin K prophylactically to a newborn infant is associated with which of the following?

a. a deficiency of factor V
b. a prolonged prothrombin time
c. development of hemorrhagic manifestations within 24 h of delivery
d. manifestations that are more severe in male than female infants
e. a greater likelihood of developing symptoms if the infant is fed cow's milk rather than breast milk

138. You are advised by the obstetrician that the mother of a baby he has delivered is a carrier of hepatitis B surface antigen (HBsAg). The most appropriate action in managing this infant would be to

a. screen the infant for HBsAg
b. isolate the infant for enteric transmission
c. screen the mother for hepatitis B "e" antigen (HBeAg)
d. administer hepatitis B immune globulin and hepatitis B vaccine
e. do nothing because transplacentally acquired antibody will prevent infection

139. Which of the following drugs given during the last 2 weeks of pregnancy is the most likely to have deleterious effects on the fetus?

a. propranolol
b. penicillin
c. aluminum hydroxide
d. phenytoin
e. heparin

140. At the time of delivery, a woman is noted to have a large volume of amniotic fluid. At 6 h of age, her baby begins regurgitating small amounts of mucus and bile-stained fluid. Physical examination of the infant is normal, and an abdominal x-ray is obtained (shown in the following figure). The most likely diagnosis of this infant's disorder is

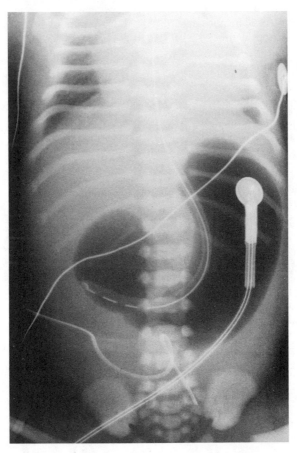

(Courtesy Susan John, M.D.)

a. gastric duplication
b. pyloric stenosis
c. esophageal atresia
d. duodenal atresia
e. midgut volvulus

Items 141–142

141. You are called to the nursery to see a baby who was noted to be jaundiced and has a serum bilirubin concentration of 13 mg/dL at 18 h of age. The baby is a 3500-g boy who was born at term to a 27-year-old primigravida 16 h after membranes ruptured. There were no prenatal complications. Breast-feeding has been well tolerated. Of the following, which is LEAST likely to be responsible for the jaundice in this baby?

a.   Rh or ABO hemolytic disease
b.   physiologic jaundice
c.   sepsis
d.   congenital spherocytic anemia
e.   glucose-6-phosphate dehydrogenase (G6PD) deficiency

142. The procedure LEAST likely to be helpful in working up this infant's jaundice is

a.   maternal and infant Rh type, blood group, and Coombs' test
b.   complete blood count, peripheral smear, and reticulocyte count
c.   total and direct bilirubin concentrations
d.   cultures
e.   liver transaminases (AST, ALT)

143. Which of the following statements about the infant in the following picture is true?

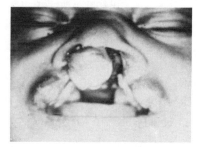

a.   parenteral alimentation is recommended to prevent aspiration
b.   surgical closure of the palatal defect should be done before 3 months of age
c.   good anatomic closure will preclude the development of speech defects
d.   recurrent otitis media and hearing loss are likely complications
e.   the chance that a sibling also would be affected is 1 in 1000

144. A 26-year-old gravida 3 woman has a history of gestational diabetes and a delivery of two previous infants at term that were greater than 4000 grams, each of whom had severe hypoglycemia. Which of the following maneuvers is least likely to reduce the chance of the next child's having hyperglycemia.

a. careful control of the maternal blood glucose levels during pregnancy
b. maternal intravenous loading with 10% glucose beginning 2 to 4 h prior to the expected time of delivery
c. careful glucose monitoring of the infant
d. early feedings of the infant
e. maintenance of the infant in a neutral thermal environment

145. A term, 4200-g female infant is delivered via cesarean section because of cephalopelvic disproportion. The amniotic fluid was clear and the infant cried almost immediately after birth. Within the first 15 min of life, however, the infant's respiratory rate increased to 80 breaths per min and she began to have intermittent grunting respirations. The infant was transferred to the level two nursery and was noted to have an oxygen saturation of 94 percent. The chest radiograph showed fluid in the fissure, overaeration, and prominent pulmonary vascular markings. The most likely diagnosis in this infant is

a. diaphragmatic hernia
b. meconium aspiration
c. pneumonia
d. idiopathic respiratory distress syndrome
e. transient tachypnea of the newborn

146. The infant in the following pictures (**A**) and (**B**) presented with hepatosplenomegaly, anemia, persistent rhinitis, and a maculopapular rash. The most likely diagnosis for this child is

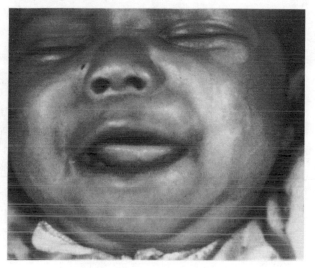

A   (Courtesy Laurence Finberg, M.D.)

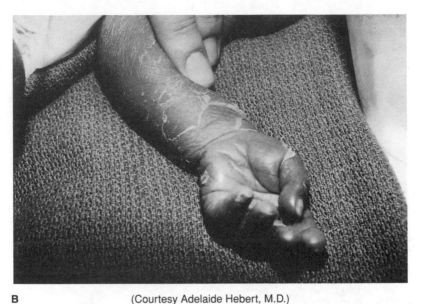

B   (Courtesy Adelaide Hebert, M.D.)

a. toxoplasmosis
b. glycogen storage disease
c. congenital hypothyroidism
d. congenital syphilis
e. cytomegalovirus disease

147. A well-appearing 3200 gram black infant is noted to have 5th finger polydactyly. The extra digit has no skeletal duplications and is attached to the rest of the hand by a thread-like soft tissue pedicle (see photograph). Appropriate treatment for this condition includes

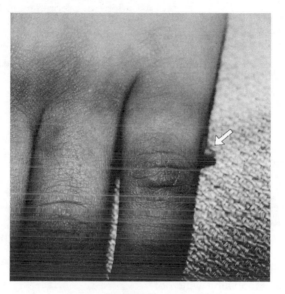

(Courtesy Adelaide Hebert, M.D.)

a.   chromosomal analysis
b.   excision of extra digit
c.   skeletal survey for other skeletal abnormalities
d.   echocardiogram
e.   renal ultrasound

148. Which of the following is a correct statement regarding neural tube defects (anencephaly, meningomyelocele)

a. the hereditary pattern is autosomal recessive
b. the prenatal diagnosis can be made by the detection of very low levels of alphafetoprotein in the amniotic fluid
c. subsequent pregnancies are not at increased risk compared to the general population
d. supplementation of maternal diet with folate leads to a decrease in incidence in this condition
e. neither environmental nor social factors have been shown to influence the incidence

149. An infant born to a heroin addict is likely to exhibit which of the following?

a. postmature dates
b. onset of withdrawal symptoms after 7 days of life
c. hyperirritability and coarse tremors
d. constipation
e. an increased incidence of hyaline membrane disease

150. A previously healthy full-term infant has several episodes of duskiness and apnea during the second day of life. Diagnostic considerations should include which of the following?

a. hemolytic anemia
b. congenital heart disease
c. idiopathic apnea
d. harlequin syndrome
e. hyperglycemia

151. In the newborn period, which of the following is an uncommon sign of meningitis?

a. lethargy
b. jaundice
c. vomiting
d. Kernig's and/or Brudzinski's sign
e. hypothermia

152. A woman gives birth to twins at 38 weeks' gestation. The first twin weighs 2800 g (6 lb, 3 oz) and has a hematocrit of 70 percent; the second twin weighs 2100 g (4 lb, 10 oz) and has a hematocrit of 40 percent. Which of the following statements is correct?

a. the second twin is at risk for developing respiratory distress, cyanosis, and congestive heart failure
b. the first twin is more likely to have hyperbilirubinemia and convulsions
c. the second twin is at risk for renal vein thrombosis
d. the second twin probably has hydramnios of the amniotic sac
e. the second twin is likely to be pale, tachycardic, and hypotensive

153. Of the following, the only one that normally rises in the infant in the first week after birth is

a. hematocrit
b. temperature
c. body weight
d. bilirubin
e. pulmonary arterial pressure

154. Oligohydramnios in a pregnant woman can indicate the presence of which of the following congenital disorders in the fetus?

a. anencephaly
b. trisomy 18
c. renal agenesis
d. duodenal atresia
e. tracheoesophageal fistula

155. A newborn infant becomes markedly jaundiced on the second day of life, and a faint petechial eruption first noted at birth is now a generalized purpuric rash. Hematologic studies for hemolytic diseases are negative. The LEAST important measure at this time would be

a. radiographic examination of the long bones
b. isolation of the infant from pregnant hospital personnel
c. a blood culture
d. lumbar puncture
e. thyroid hormone assay

DIRECTIONS: Each group of questions below consists of lettered options followed by numbered items. For each numbered item, select the appropriate lettered option(s). Each lettered option may be used once, more than once, or not at all. **Choose exactly the number of options indicated following each item.**

Items 156–159

For each jaundiced infant described below, select the lettered curve on the graph that best represents the expected course of that infant's serum bilirubin.

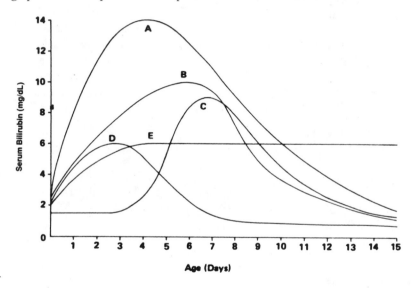

156. A premature neonate who is otherwise normal (**SELECT 1 CURVE**)

157. A full-term neonate who is found to have septicemia on day 4 (**SELECT 1 CURVE**)

158. A full-term neonate with hypothyroidism (**SELECT 1 CURVE**)

159. A full-term neonate who has erythroblastosis fetalis (**SELECT 1 CURVE**)

Items 160–163

Amniocentesis is a valuable tool for prenatal diagnosis and treatment of several diseases. Match the disease with the appropriate test.

a. alpha-fetoprotein
b. lecithin/sphingomyelin ratio (L/S)
c. karyotype
d. enzyme determination
e. bilirubin

160. Neural tube defect
(SELECT 1 TEST)

161. Trisomy 21
(SELECT 1 TEST)

162. Respiratory distress syndrome
(SELECT 1 TEST)

163. Tay-Sachs disease
(SELECT 1 TEST)

Items 164–167

Blood samples of a 3-day-old full-term infant are sent for screening to identify diseases that would have serious permanent consequences without prompt and appropriate treatment. Match the disease with the treatment.

a. special diet
b. hormone therapy
c. vitamin therapy
d. antibiotic prophylaxis
e. sunlight

164. Galactosemia
(SELECT 1 TREATMENT)

165. Phenylketonuria
(SELECT 1 TREATMENT)

166. Biotinidase deficiency
(SELECT 1 TREATMENT)

167. Hypothyroidism
(SELECT 1 TREATMENT)

Items 168–171

For each description of a congenital anomaly that follows, select the major abnormality with which it is most likely to be associated.

a. deafness
b. seizures
c. Wilms' tumor
d. congestive heart failure
e. optic glioma

168. Nonfamilial bilateral absence of the iris (aniridia)
(SELECT 1 ABNORMALITY)

169. Heterochromia of the iris, broad nasal root, fusion of the eyebrows, and white forelock
(SELECT 1 ABNORMALITY)

170. Flat capillary vascular malformation over the anterior scalp and one side of the face
(SELECT 1 ABNORMALITY)

171. Hypopigmented oval macules on the skin of the trunk and extremities
(SELECT 1 ABNORMALITY)

Items 172–174

For each description of head injury that follows, select the major abnormality with which it is most likely to be associated.

a. intraventricular hemorrhage
b. caput succedaneum
c. subdural hemorrhage
d. subarachnoid hemorrhage
e. cephalhematoma

172. One-day-old healthy infant with a superficial swelling over the right parietotemporal region that does not cross the suture lines
(SELECT 1 ABNORMALITY)

173. Six-month-old comatose infant with multiple broken bones in various stages of healing, bulging anterior fontanelle, and retinal hemorrhages
(SELECT 1 ABNORMALITY)

174. Previous premature infant born at 27-weeks' gestation and now 6 months of age presenting with macrocephaly and hydrocephalus on ultrasonogram
(SELECT 1 ABNORMALITY)

THE NEWBORN INFANT

Answers

108. The answer is d. (*Behrman, 16/e, pp. 328, 441, 531, 1580. McMillan, 3/e, pp. 356–358, 1600, 2228, 2230. Rudolph, 20/e, pp. 248–251, 297–299, 421, 1371–1372.*) Fetal alcohol syndrome is a preventable cause of birth defects. Prenatal exposure to ethanol is the cause. Findings include microcephaly, small palpebral fissures, short nose, smooth philtrum, thin upper lip, ptosis, microphthalmia, cleft lip and palate, and central nervous system abnormalities including mental retardation (average IQ = 67).

Common findings with trisomy 21 include protruding tongue, Brushfield's spots, redundant neck skin, mental retardation, brachycephaly, upslanting palpebral fissures, epicanthal folds, flat face, small ears, cardiac abnormalities (especially ventricular septal defect or endocardial cushing defect), palmar creases, and clinodactyly of the 5th digit.

Dilantin exposure causes mid face hypoplasia, low nasal bridge, ocular hypertelorism, and accentuated cupid's bow of the upper lip. Other features include cleft lip and palate, growth retardation, mental deficiency, distal phalangeal hyperplasia, cardiovascular anamolies, and skeletal defects.

In 85 percent of patients with Alport's syndrome, an X-linked dominant form of inheritance is found; about 15 percent are autosomal recessive. All cause hematuria and progressive nephritis. Other findings include deafness and ocular defects.

Infants of diabetic mothers have an increased chance of congenital heart disease, caudal regression syndrome, a small left colon, being large for gestation age, and a number of biochemical abnormalities.

109. The answer is d. (*Behrman, 16/e pp. 513–517. McMillan, 3/e, 197–206. Rudolph, 20/e, pp. 1133–1137.*) Significant unconjugated bilirubin levels in serum in full-term newborn infants can lead to diffusion of bilirubin into brain tissue and to neurologic damage. Sulfisoxazole and other drugs compete with bilirubin for binding sites on albumin; therefore, the presence of these drugs can cause dislocation of bilirubin to tissues, not increased affinity. Metabolic acidosis also reduces binding of bilirubin and neonatal sepsis interrupts the blood-brain barrier, thus allowing diffusion of bilirubin into the brain. Administration of phenobarbital has been used to induce glucuronyl transferase in newborn infants and can reduce, rather than exacerbate, neonatal jaundice. Other factors that reduce the amount of unconjugated bilirubin bound to albumin (and therefore cause an increase in free unconjugated bilirubin) include hypoalbuminemia and certain compounds (e.g., nonesterified fatty acids, which are elevated during cold stress) that compete with bilirubin for albumin binding sites.

110. The answer is c. (*Behrman, 16/e, pp. 495, 1258–1259[C1]. Rudolph 20/e, pp. 954–955.*) It is important to make the diagnosis of choanal atresia quickly in that it responds to treatment but can be lethal if unrecognized and untreated. Most neonates are obligate nose breathers because they cannot breathe adequately through their mouths. Infants with choanal atresia have increased breathing difficulty during feeding and sleeping and improve when crying. A variety of temporizing measures to maintain an open airway have been used, including oropharyngeal airways, positioning, tongue fixation, and endotracheal intubation, but surgical correction with placement of nasal tubes is most effective. The diagnosis can be made by failure to pass a catheter through the nose to the pharynx.

111. The answer is e. (*Behrman, 16/e, pp. 974, 977, 1088. McMillan, 3/e, pp. 436–437. Rudolph, 20/e, pp. 684–686.*) Varicella-zoster immunoglobulin (VZIG) should be administered to the infant immediately after delivery if the mother had the onset of varicella within 5 days prior to delivery, and immediately upon diagnosis if her chickenpox started within 2 days after delivery. If untreated, about half of these infants will develop serious varicella as early as 1 day of age. If a normal full-term newborn is exposed to chickenpox 2 or more days postnatally, VZIG and isolation are not necessary because these babies appear to be at no greater risk for complications than older children. Acyclovir is not approved for use in early infancy.

112. The answer is b. (*Behrman, 16/e, p. 164. McMillan, 3/e, p. 470. Rudolph, 20/e, pp. 22–23.*) A normal 2-week-old infant has a basal caloric expenditure of about 65 cal/kg per day. Adding calories for activity and growth brings the caloric requirement to about 110 cal/kg. A 3.5-kg infant, therefore, requires about 385 cal in the diet per day. Standard infant formulas have a caloric density of 0.67 cal/mL, so it would take about 575 mL of infant formula per day to supply adequate calories for this infant. For the infant in question, 60 mL four times a day (240 mL per day) is less than half of the amount that the infant needs and should be of concern. The other factors in the question are normal for the infant's age.

113. The answer is a. *(Behrman, 16/e pp. 493–495. McMillan, 3/e, pp. 179–180, 235–7. Rudolph 20/e, pp. 1882–1884.)* During a period of asphyxia, the resulting hypoxemia, acidosis, and poor perfusion can damage a neonate's brain, heart, kidney, liver, and lungs. The resulting clinical abnormalities include cerebral edema, irritability, seizures, cardiomegaly, heart failure, renal failure, poor liver function, disseminated intravascular coagulopathy, and respiratory distress syndrome. There can be excessively high pulmonary arterial pressure at the same time systemic blood pressure begins to fall, resulting in a persistent right-to-left shunt across a patent ductus arteriosus or foramen ovale.

114. The answer is a. *(Behrman, 16/e, pp. 981–983. McMillan, 3/e, pp. 429 433. Rudolph, 20/e, pp. 629–633.)* Cytomegalic inclusion disease is the most common congenital viral infection. In the United States, 20 percent to 90 percent of women of childbearing age have serologic evidence of a past infection with CMV. Symptomatic congenital disease usually occurs when a mother has a primary CMV infection in the first trimester of pregnancy. Many of these babies die and those who survive are severely affected. In the event of reactivation of CMV infection during pregnancy, maternal IgG, passed transplacentally, protects the infant from serious infection. Although most infants infected during this secondary maternal infection are asymptomatic, about 10 percent of them eventually manifest hearing and neurologic problems. Some recommend keeping a child with congenital CMV infection away from susceptible pregnant, or about to become pregnant, women because CMV excretion can persist for months to years; at the very least, good hand washing should be instituted. If infected shortly after birth, the younger sibling will probably be asymptomatic since he or she has maternal IgG in the circulation. CMV is primarily an occult infection. Twenty percent to eighty percent of toddlers in day-care centers acquire CMV and shed it in saliva and urine for years. The "gold or criterion standard" for diagnosis is a urine viral culture for CMV.

115. The answer is b. *(Behrman, 16/e, pp. 526–527, 1101. McMillan, 3/e, p. 360. Rudolph, 20/e, p. 1042.)* Hematemesis and melena are not uncommon in the neonatal period, especially if gross placental bleeding has occurred at the time of delivery. The diagnostic procedure that should be done first is the Apt test, which differentiates fetal from adult hemoglobin in a bloody specimen. If the blood in an affected infant's gastric contents or stool is maternal in origin, further workup of the infant is obviated.

116. The answer is d. *(Behrman, 16/e pp. 464–467. McMillan, 3/e, p. 152. Rudolph, 20/e, pp. 203–205.)* Baseline variability with or without periodic acceleration of the fetal heart rate is a sign of fetal well-being. Increasing baseline variability (saltatory pattern) can represent early compromise of fetal oxygenation. The early deceleration pattern is due to head compression and is not a sign of fetal distress. The variable deceleration pattern indicates compression of the umbilical cord. The late deceleration pattern, if repetitive, signifies fetal hypoxemia. Either of these last two patterns in association with loss of baseline variability is a sign of severe fetal compromise.

117. The answer is a. *(Behrman, 16/e, pp. 545, 548–549, 802–806, 885–897, 996–998, 1041, 1054–1062, 1922. McMillan, 3/e, pp. 427–454, 978–980, 1099. Rudolph, 20/e, pp. 629–633, 653, 681–683, 769–770.)* The newborn whose mother acquired her primary infection with *Toxoplasma gondii* early in pregnancy will be severely affected. Later transmission during pregnancy occurs more often, but babies so infected are only mildly ill or even asymptomatic. The acronym TORCH refers to toxoplasmosis, other congenital infections, rubella, CMV, and herpes simplex. The "other congenital infections" include syphilis, varicella, hepatitis, and parvovirus, HIV, enterovirus, listeria, and coxsackie infections. There is no such thing as a "TORCH titer." In making a diagnosis of a congenital infection, each disease must be investigated separately. Rubella, CMV, and herpesvirus can be cultured shortly after birth. Sequential IgG levels are helpful in diagnosing rubella and toxoplasmosis. Specific IgM titers are diagnostic in rubella infections but false negative results occur in toxoplasmosis. Many clinical laboratories are not equipped to perform IgM assays. Rotavirus has not been shown to cause congenital infection. Group B streptococcus causes neonatal infections but typically group A streptococcus does not. *Mycobacterium tuberculosis* is potentially acquired in the newborn period, but rarely is it transmitted across the placenta. Typically, *Trichomonas* does not cause a congenital infection.

118. The answer is b. (*Behrman, 16/e pp. 480–482. McMillan, 3/e, pp. 146–148. Rudolph, 20/e, pp. 235–237.*) It is usually impossible with any combination of parenteral and enteral nutrition to match what the infant would have accumulated in utero. The average, healthy, low-birth-weight infant of this size requires a daily intake of calcium of about 200 mg/kg. Breast milk has much less calcium (and phosphorus) than do commercial formulas. The breast milk can be supplemented with calcium, or it can be mixed with commercial formulas designed for the premature infant. Breast milk promotes gut maturation and prevents intestinal atrophy induced by lack of enteral feeding. Breast milk, however, is likely to have insufficient calcium and phosphorus for catch-up growth.

119. The answer is d. (*McMillan, 3/e, p. 218. Rudolph, 20/e, pp. 225, 230–231.*) A room temperature of 24°C (approximately 75°F) provides a cold environment for newborn infants. Aside from the fact that these infants emerge from a warm 37.6°C (99.5°F) intrauterine environment, at birth, infants (and especially preterm infants) are wet, have a relatively large surface area for their weight, and have little subcutaneous fat. Within minutes of delivery, the infants are likely to become pale or blue and their body temperatures will drop. In order to bring body temperature back to normal, they must increase their metabolic rate; ventilation, in turn, must increase proportionally to ensure an adequate oxygen supply. Because a preterm infant is likely to have respiratory problems and be unable to oxygenate adequately, lactate can accumulate and lead to a metabolic acidosis. Infants rarely shiver in response to a need to increase heat production.

120. The answer is b. (*Behrman, 16/e pp. 521–525. McMillan, 3/e, p. 361. Rudolph, 20/e, p. 1200.*) If a mother is O-positive and her baby is A-positive, the baby has a chance of developing hemolytic disease. Hemolytic disease and jaundice caused by a major blood-group incompatibility are usually less severe than with Rh incompatibility. Although the hematocrit of affected infants usually is normal, elevation of the reticulocyte count and the presence of nucleated red blood cells and microspherocytes in the blood smear provide evidence of hemolysis. In comparison with hemolytic disease caused by Rh incompatibility, where it is usually strongly positive, major blood-group incompatibility is often associated with a direct Coombs' test that is frequently weakly positive.

121. The answer is a. (*Behrman, 16/e pp. 475–477. McMillan, 3/e, pp. 206–209. Rudolph, 20/e, pp. 244–248.*) Small-for-dates infants are subject to a different set of complications than preterm infants whose size is appropriate for gestational age. The small-for-dates infants have a higher incidence of major congenital anomalies and are at increased risk for future growth retardation, especially if length and head circumference as well as weight are small for gestational age. Also more common are neonatal asphyxia and the meconium aspiration syndrome, which can lead to pneumothorax, pneumomediastinum, or pulmonary hemorrhage. These, rather than hyaline membrane disease, are the major pulmonary problems in these infants. Because neonatal symptomatic hypoglycemia is more commonly found in small-for-dates infants, careful blood glucose monitoring and early feeding are appropriate precautions. Normal or elevated hematocrit is also more common in these infants.

122. The answer is a. (*Behrman, 16/e, pp. 497–498. McMillan, 3/e, pp. 265–266. Rudolph, 20/e, pp. 1593–1595.*) Apneic episodes are characterized by an absence of respirations for more than 20 sec and may be accompanied by bradycardia and cyanosis. A large number of conditions can cause apnea. Periods of apnea are generally thought to be secondary to an incompletely developed respiratory center, particularly when they are seen, as is common, associated with prematurity. Although seizures, hypoglycemia, and pulmonary disease accompanied by hypoxia can lead to apnea, these causes are less likely in the infant described, given that no unusual movements occur during the apneic spells, that the blood sugar level is more than 40 mg/dL, and that the child appears well between episodes. Periodic breathing, a common pattern of respiration in low-birth-weight babies, is characterized by recurrent breathing pauses of 3 to 10 sec.

123–124. The answers are 123–c, 124–c. (*Behrman, 16/e pp. 510, 1698–1703. McMillan, 3/e, pp. 354–355, 1806–1809. Rudolph, 20/e, 1757–1761.*) The main thrust of both questions is directed at the need for speed in the diagnosis and treatment of congenital hypothyroidism because the earlier treatment is started with thyroid hormone, the better the prognosis for intellectual function. Time should not be spent in exhaustive investigation. Regardless of the reason for the hypothyroidism, treatment with thyroid hormone is indicated. If it turns out that the initial diagnosis was erroneous, little harm will be done by treating an infant with a physiologic dose of thyroid hormone for a few days. Waiting for laboratory tests or x-rays to be performed, interpreted, and probably repeated is inappropriate if this will delay treatment. Eventually, they should be done, along with an evaluation of the mother's immune status, her health history, and a complete family history looking for one of the many known, although relatively rare, causes of congenital hypothyroidism. Thyroid dysgenesis is found in 90 percent of the cases. Neonatal screening for hypothyroidism has allowed for the much earlier diagnosis of hypothyroidism, resulting in improvement of prognosis, so that frank cretinism is now quite rare.

125–126. The answers are 125–c, 126–c. *(Behrman, 16/e, p. 491. McMillan, 3/e, pp. 164, 2122. Rudolph, 20/e, pp. 214–215, 224, 1939.)* In a difficult delivery in which traction is applied to the head and neck, several injuries, including all those listed in the question, may occur. Erb-Duchenne paralysis affects the fifth and sixth cervical nerves; the affected arm cannot be abducted or externally rotated at the shoulder, and the forearm cannot be supinated. Injury to the seventh and eighth cervical and first thoracic nerves (Klumpke's paralysis) results in palsy of the hand and also can produce Horner's syndrome. Fractures in the upper limb are not associated with a characteristic posture, and passive movement usually elicits pain. Spinal injury causes complete paralysis below the level of injury.

When paralysis of an upper extremity from injury to the brachial plexus is found in a neonate, injury to the phrenic nerve should also be suspected because the nerve roots are close together and can be injured concurrently. The paralyzed diaphragm can be noted to remain elevated on a chest x-ray taken during deep inspiration when it will contrast with the opposite normal diaphragm in its lower normal position, but on expiration this asymmetry cannot be seen. On inspiration not only is breathing impaired since the paralyzed diaphragm does not contract, but the negative pressure generated by the intact diaphragm pulls the mediastinum toward the normal side, impairing ventilation further. The diagnosis can easily be made by fluoroscopy, where these characteristic movements on inspiration and expiration can be seen. Rarely, both diaphragms can be paralyzed, producing much more severe ventilatory impairment. Fortunately, these injuries frequently improve spontaneously.

127. The answer is a. *(Behrman, 16/e, pp. 525–526. McMillan, 3/e, pp. 141, 240–245, 362–363. Rudolph, 20/e, pp. 200, 252–255, 1957.)* An infant of

2100 g at 38 weeks would be considered small for gestational age (SGA), a not uncommon consequence of maternal toxemia. Pregnancy-induced hypertension can produce a decrease in uteroplacental blood flow and areas of placental infarction. This can result in fetal nutritional deprivation and intermittent fetal hypoxemia, with a decrease in glycogen storage and a relative erythrocytosis, respectively. Hence, neonatal hypoglycemia and polycythemia are common clinical findings in these infants. A blood glucose level of 30 mg/dL in a full-term infant, however, is probably normal during the first postnatal day and an infant is very unlikely to have a convulsion as a result of a level of 38 mg. Serum calcium levels usually decline during the first 2 to 3 postnatal days, but will only be considered abnormally low in a term infant when they fall below 7.5 to 8 mg/dL. Neonatal hypermagnesemia is common in an infant whose mother has received $MgSO_4$ therapy, but is usually asymptomatic or produces decreased muscle tone or floppiness. A persistent venous hematocrit of greater than 65 percent in a neonate is regarded as polycythemia and will be accompanied by an increase in blood viscosity. Manifestations of the "hyperviscosity syndrome" include tremulousness or jitteriness that can progress to seizure activity because of sludging of blood in the cerebral microcirculation or frank thrombus formation, renal vein thrombosis, necrotizing enterocolitis, and tachypnea. Therapy by partial exchange transfusion with albumin is probably more likely to be useful if performed prophylactically before significant symptoms have developed.

128. The answer is b. (*Behrman, 16/e p. 495. McMillan, 3/e, pp. 173–178. Rudolph, 20/e, pp. 238–243.*) In the description provided, the most likely cause of the neonatal depression is maternal analgesic narcotic drug administration. While controlling the pain of the delivery in the mother, use of narcotics can result in depression of the newborn via crossing of the placenta. Appropriate first steps in the management of this infant (after managing the ABCs of airway, breathing, and circulation) is the administration of naloxone, 0.1 mg/kg, IM, IV, or intratracheal. The other possibilities are unlikely given the clinical information provided.

129. The answer is a. (*Behrman, 16/e pp. 505–506. McMillan, 3/e, pp. 173–178. Rudolph, 20/e, pp. 238–243.*) Infants who are postmature (more than 42 weeks' gestation) and show evidence of chronic placental insufficiency (low birth weight for gestational age and wasted appearance) have a higher-than-average chance of being asphyxiated, and passage of meconium into the amniotic fluid thus places these infants at risk for meconium aspiration. To prevent or minimize this risk, these infants should have immediate nasopharyngeal suction as their heads are delivered. Immediately after delivery and before initiation of respiration, their tracheas should be carefully and thoroughly suctioned through an endotracheal tube under direct vision with a laryngoscope. Afterward, appropriate resuscitative measures should be undertaken to establish adequate ventilation and circulation. Artificial ventilation performed before tracheal suction could force meconium into smaller airways.

130. The answer is b. *(Behrman, 16/e pp. 1911–1914. McMillan, 3/e, pp. 668–669. Rudolph 214, 2078.)* The time of onset of symptoms is somewhat helpful in the diagnosis of ophthalmia neonatorum. Chemical conjunctivitis is a self-limited condition that presents within 6 to 12 h of birth as a consequence of silver nitrate prophylaxis. Gonococcal conjunctivitis has its onset within 2 to 5 days after birth and is the most serious of the bacterial infections. Prompt and aggressive topical treatment and systemic antibiotics are indicated to prevent serious complications. Parents should be treated to avoid the risk to the child of reinfection. Silver nitrate is believed by some to be ineffective prophylaxis against chlamydial conjunctivitis, which occurs 5 to 14 days after birth. To avoid the risk of chlamydial pneumonia, treatment with systemic antibiotics is indicated for the infant as well as both parents.

131. The answer is b. *(Behrman, 16/e, pp. 498–505. McMillan, 3/e, pp. 254–258. Rudolph, 20/e, pp. 1598–1605.)* For the child described in the question, prematurity and the clinical picture presented make the diagnosis of hyaline membrane disease likely. In this disease, lung compliance is reduced; lung volume also is reduced and a significant right-to-left shunt of blood can occur. Some of the shunt can result from a patent ductus arteriosus or foramen ovale, and some can be due to shunting in the lung. Minute ventilation is higher than normal and affected infants must work harder in order to sustain adequate breathing.

132. The answer is e. *(Behrman, 16/e, p. 1799. McMillan, 3/e, pp. 164, 760, 1910–1917. Rudolph, 20/e, pp. 218–223.)* Normal term neonates demonstrate a large number of reflex patterns that are mediated by the brainstem or spinal cord. The glabellar tap response (blinking of eyelids in response to a tap on the glabella) develops between 32 and 35 weeks' gestation. The scarf sign is associated with the normal relative hypotonicity of the preterm infant. The Moro response may remain incomplete for a varying period, but should always be complete (including the embrace) by term; it is too variable to be used for evaluating gestational age. The plantar response is not a true Babinski response and should not be referred to as such. Serpentine tongue movements are always abnormal.

Other reflexes seen in the term infant include the sucking and rooting reflexes; the stepping reflex, by which movements of forward progression are elicited on a flat surface; the placing reflex, which produces leg flexion; and the palmar and plantar grasps, which are induced by slight pressure on the palms and soles. The parachute reaction, a protective reflex characterized by extension of the arms and hands when an infant in the prone position is brought sharply toward a firm surface, does not appear until the age of 9 months. The parachute reaction persists for life, whereas the other primitive reflexes disappear in the early months.

133. The answer is c. *(Behrman, 16/e, pp. 1753–1755. McMillan, 3/e, pp. 1775, 2231. Rudolph, 20/e, pp. 215, 1782–1785.)* Turner's syndrome is a genetic disorder; the 45,XO karyotype is the most common. At birth, affected infants have low weights, short stature, edema over the dorsum of the hands and feet, and loose skin folds at the nape of the neck. Some other findings with this syndrome include sexual infantalism, streak gonads, atypical faces, shield chest, low hairline, coarctation of the aorta, hypertension, bicuspic aortic valve, high palate, and horseshoe kidney. Coarse, tremulous movements accompanied by ankle clonus; vascular instability as evidenced, for example, by a harlequin color change (a transient, longitudinal division of a body into red and pale halves); softness of parietal bones at the vertex (craniotabes); and a liver that is palpable down to 2 cm below the costal margin are all findings often demonstrated by normal infants and are of no diagnostic significance in the clinical situation presented.

134. The answer is b. *(Behrman, 16/e, pp. 455. 1971–1972. McMillan, 3/e, pp. 372, 682, 711. Rudolph, 20/e, pp. 212, 902.)* Mongolian spots are bluish-gray lesions located over the buttock, lower back, and occasionally, the extensor surfaces of the extremities. They are common in blacks, Asians, and Latin Americans. They tend to disappear by 1 to 2 years of age, although those on the extremities may not fully resolve. Child abuse is unlikely to present with bruises alone; children frequently present with more extensive injuries. Subcutaneous fat necrosis is usually found as a sharply demarcated, hard lesion on the cheeks, buttocks, and limbs. The lesion usually is red. Hemophilia and vitamin K deficiency rarely present with subcutaneous lesions as described and are more likely to present as a bleeding episode.

135. The answer is c. *(Behrman, 16/e, pp. 1231–1233. McMillan, 3/e, pp 177, 217–218, 222. Rudolph, 20/e, pp. 215, 1588–1590.)* Diaphragmatic hernia occurs with the transmittal of abdominal contents across a congenital or traumatic defect in the diaphragm. In the newborn, this condition results in profound respiratory distress with significant mortality. Prenatal diagnosis is common and when found, necessitates that the birth take place at a tertiary level center. In the neonate, respiratory failure in the first hours of life, a scaphoid abdomen, and presence of bowel sounds in the chest are common findings. Intensive respiratory support including mechanical ventilation and extracorporeal membrane oxygenation (ECMO) has increased survival. Mortality can be as high as 50 percent despite aggressive treatment.

136. The answer is d. *(Behrman, 16/e, pp. 1122–1123. McMillan, 3/e, pp. 309–310. Rudolph, 20/e, pp. 215, 402.)* Abdominal distention, choking, drooling, and coughing associated with feedings are symptoms of esophageal anomalies. The anomaly illustrated by figure **D** is the most common; that of figure **A** can be diagnosed after repeated episodes of pneumonia. The anomalies in figures **E** and **C** are associated with all the same symptoms except abdominal distention, which cannot develop because air cannot enter the gastrointestinal tract. **B** and **C** are the least common; in these, the upper esophageal segment is connected directly to the trachea and massive entry of fluid into the lungs occurs.

VATER syndrome, a complex of cardiovascular malformations, skeletal malformations, and renal abnormalities, has tracheoesophageal fistula as a common finding.

137. The answer is b. *(Behrman, 16/e, pp. 459, 526. McMillan, 3/e, pp. 367, 1487–1488. Rudolph, 20/e, p. 1249.)* Failure to give vitamin K prophylactically to newborn infants is associated with a decline in the levels of vitamin K-dependent coagulation factors. In less than 1 percent of infants (but especially those fed human breast milk), the levels reached are low enough to produce classic hemorrhagic manifestations on the second to seventh day of life. These manifestations include melena, hematuria, and bleeding from the circumcision; intracranial hemorrhage and hypovolemic shock are serious complications. Diagnosis of this condition is indicated by a prolonged prothrombin time, which reflects inadequate concentrations of factors II, VII, IX, and X.

138. The answer is d. *(Behrman, 16/e, pp. 771–773, 775–776. McMillan, 3/e, pp. 447–449, 1724–1725. Rudolph, 20/e, pp. 227, 648–650.)* The infant of a mother who is a carrier of hepatitis B surface antigen has a significant risk of acquiring infection. This usually occurs at the time of delivery, but infection can also be acquired during pregnancy and postnatally. A small percentage of infected neonates develop acute icteric hepatitis, but the majority remain asymptomatic. Of these infected asymptomatic infants, 80 percent or more will develop chronic antigenemia, the long-term consequences of which are chronic liver disease and possibly, hepatocellular carcinoma. Combined passive-active immunoprophylaxis in the form of immune globulin and hepatitis B vaccine affords protection not only from immediate perinatal infection but also from infection that may be acquired as a result of continued exposure in the household of a chronic carrier.

Immunization is indicated regardless of the presence of hepatitis B "e" antigen (HBeAg) in the mother. Although the presence of HBeAg, especially in the absence of antibody to HBeAg, is associated with high rates of transmission to neonates, any woman positive for hepatitis B surface antigen (HbsAg) is potentially infectious. It is not necessary to isolate infants born to carriers of HBsAg and screening of neonates for HBsAg is not indicated. Testing for HBsAg and anti-HBsAg at least 1 month after the third dose of hepatitis B vaccine will determine the efficacy of these measures.

139. The answer is a. *(Behrman, 16/e, pp. 467–469. McMillan, 3/e, pp. 137–139. Rudolph, 20/e, pp. 421, 1832.)* The effect of a drug on the fetus is determined by the nature of the drug and by the timing and degree of exposure. Heparin does not cross the placental barrier and does not appear to directly affect the fetus once pregnancy is well established. Phenytoin may cause birth defects when given during the first trimester. Penicillin and aluminum hydroxide have not been found to affect the fetus. Propranolol, which may cause growth retardation when given throughout pregnancy, diminishes the ability of an asphyxiated infant to increase heart rate and cardiac output. It has also been associated with hypoglycemia and apnea.

140. The answer is d. *(Behrman, 16/e, pp. 1133–1134. McMillan, 3/e, p. 312. Rudolph, 20/e, p. 1069.)* The findings of polyhydramnios signal high intestinal obstruction, signs of which include abdominal distention and early and repeated regurgitation. Distention usually is not present as vomiting keeps the intestine decompressed. The bile-stained vomitus of the infant places the obstruction distal to the ampulla of Vater, eliminating esophageal atresia and pyloric stenosis from consideration. The "double bubble" sign on the x-ray is characteristic of duodenal atresia, which is compatible with the history. Midgut volvulus, which may obstruct the bowel in the area of the duodenojejunal junction, most often produces signs after an affected infant is 3 or 4 days old with acute onset of bilious vomitus. Gastric duplication does not usually produce intestinal obstruction; a cystic mass may be palpated on abdominal examination. Patients with duodenal atresia should be examined closely for evidence of other conditions such as Down syndrome or heart disease.

141–142. The answers are 141–b, 142–e. *(Behrman, 16/e, pp. 513–517. McMillan, 3/e, pp. 197–206. Rudolph, 20/e, pp. 210–211, 1133–1136, 1193–1196.)* The development of jaundice in a healthy full-term baby may be considered the result of a normal physiologic process if the time of onset and duration of the jaundice and the pattern of serially determined serum concentrations of bilirubin are in conformity with currently accepted safe criteria. Physiologic jaundice becomes apparent on the second or third day of life, peaks to levels no higher than about 12 mg/dL on the fourth or fifth day, and disappears by the end of the week. The rate of rise is less than 5 mg/dL per 24 h and levels of conjugated bilirubin do not exceed about 1 mg/dL. Concern about neonatal jaundice relates to the risk of the neurotoxic effects of unconjugated bilirubin. The precise level and duration of exposure necessary to produce toxic effects are not known, but bilirubin encephalopathy, or kernicterus, is rare in term infants whose bilirubin level is kept below 18 to 20 mg/dL. Certain risk factors affecting premature or sick newborns increase their susceptibility to kernicterus at much lower levels of bilirubin. The diagnosis of physiologic jaundice is made by excluding other causes of hyperbilirubinemia by means of history, physical examination, and laboratory determinations. Jaundice appearing in the first 24 h is usually a feature of hemolytic states and is accompanied by an indirect hyperbilirubinemia, reticulocytosis, and evidence of red-cell destruction on smear. In the absence of blood group or Rh incompatibility, congenital hemolytic states (e.g., spherocytic anemia) or G6PD deficiency should be considered. With infection, hemolytic and hepatotoxic factors are reflected in the increased levels of both direct and indirect bilirubin.

Studies should include maternal and infant Rh types and blood groups and Coombs' tests to detect blood group or Rh incompatibility and sensitization. Measurements of total and direct bilirubin concentrations help to determine the level of production of bilirubin and the presence of conjugated hyperbilirubinemia. Hematocrit and reticulocyte count provide information as to the degree of hemolysis and anemia, and a complete blood count screens for the possibility of sepsis and the need for cultures. Examination of the blood smear is useful in differentiating common hemolytic disorders. Except for determinations of total and direct bilirubin, tests of liver function are not particularly helpful in establishing the cause of early-onset jaundice. Transient elevations of transaminases (AST and ALT) related to the trauma of delivery and to hypoxia have been noted. Biliary atresia and neonatal hepatitis can be accompanied by elevated levels of transaminase but characteristically present as chronic cholestatic jaundice with mixed hyperbilirubinemia after the first week of life.

143. The answer is d. (*Behrman, 16e, pp. 1111–1113. McMillan, 3/e, pp. 391–394, 2253, 2256. Rudolph, 20/e, pp. 411, 413, 415, 962–964.*) The infant pictured has bilateral cleft lip and palate. This defect occurs in about 4 percent of the siblings of affected infants; its incidence in the general population is 1 in 1000. Evaluation for other structural and chromosomal abnormalities is indicated. Although affected infants are likely to have feeding problems initially, these problems usually can be overcome by feeding in a propped-up position and using special nipples. Complications include recurrent otitis media and hearing loss as well as speech defects, which may be present despite good anatomic closure. Repair of a cleft lip usually is performed within the first 2 to 3 months of life; the palate is repaired later, usually between the ages of 6 months and 5 years.

144. The answer is b. (*Behrman, 16/e, pp. 441, 532–533. McMillan, 3/e, pp. 346–347, 356–358. Rudolph, 20/e, pp. 248–251.*) Glucose loading of the mother will result in fetal hyperglycemia, which causes insulin release and reactive hypoglycemia. Careful medical support of the antepartum woman diminishes the hypertrophy of the fetal islet cells. Careful monitoring of the infant with early feeding or intravenous infusion of glucose can prevent hypoglycemia. A neutral thermal environment diminishes glucose consumption and, therefore, helps with glucose homeostasis.

145. The answer is e. *(Behrman, 16e, p505. McMillan, 3/e, p. 259. Rudolph, 20/e, 1597–1598.)* Transient tachypnea of the newborn is usually seen after a normal vaginal or especially after a cesarean delivery. These patients have tachypnea, retractions, grunting, and sometimes, cyanosis. The chest examination is usually normal; the chest radiograph demonstrates prominent pulmonary vascular markings with fluid in the fissures and hyperexpansion (flat diaphragms). Therapy is supportive with maintenance of normal oxygen saturation. Resolution usually occurs in the first 3 days of life.

146. The answer is d. *(Behrman, 16e, pp. 903–907. McMillan, 3/e, pp. 438–442. Rudolph, 20/e, pp. 610–612, 887.)* The clinical presentation of congenital syphilis is varied. Many newborns appear normal at birth and continue to be asymptomatic for the first few weeks or months of life. Most untreated infants will develop a skin lesion, the usual one being an infiltrative, maculopapular peeling rash that is most prominent on the face, palms, and soles. Involvement of the nasal mucous membranes causes rhinitis with a resultant serous and occasionally purulent, blood-tinged discharge (snuffles). This, as well as scrapings from the skin lesions, contains abundant viable treponemes. Hepatosplenomegaly and lymphadenopathy are common and early jaundice is a manifestation of syphilitic hepatitis. Among the later manifestations, or stigmata, of congenital syphilis is interstitial keratitis, which is an acute inflammation of the cornea that begins in early childhood (most commonly between 6 and 14 years of age). Interstitial keratitis represents the response of the tissue to earlier sensitization. Findings include marked photophobia, lacrimation, corneal haziness, and eventual scarring.

147. The answer is b. *(Behrman, 16/e, p. 2093. McMillan, 3/e, p. 2123. Rudolph, 20/e, p. 2133.)* Fifth finger polydactly is 10 times more common in black than in white children. This finding in otherwise healthy black children should raise no special concern. In a white child, careful examination of the cardiac system is warranted.

148. The answer is d. *(Behrman, 16e, pp. 1803–1806. McMillan, 3/e, pp. 156, 223–224. Rudolph, 20/e, pp. 281, 412, 1181.)* Diseases that are due to defects in a single gene are designated as autosomal or X linked depending on whether the affected gene is located on an autosome or an X chromosome. Genetically determined diseases that are multifactorial in origin (i.e., neural tube defects) do not conform to the mendelian pattern of inheritance but exhibit a variable outcome that reflects the interaction between a particular genotype and an environment. The relatives of persons with diseases of multifactorial origin have an increased risk of having similar abnormalities. The recurrence risk for most single primary defects of multifactorial inheritance (e.g., neural tube defects) is increased with each child affected. This increased risk forms the basis for assuming that genetic factors play a role in the occurrence of these abnormalities. Other factors, such as race, sex, and ethnic and racial background, influence the frequency with which an abnormality of multifactorial inheritance occurs in relatives. The prenatal diagnosis of neural tube defects (anencephaly and meningomyelocele) can be made by the detection of elevated levels of alpha-fetoprotein in the amniotic fluid. To reduce the risk of neural tube defects, it is now recommended that all women capable of becoming pregnant take 4 mg of folic acid daily.

149. The answer is c. *(Behrman, 16/e, p. 530. Rudolph, 20/e, p. 192.)* Infants born to narcotic addicts are more likely than other children to exhibit a variety of problems, including perinatal complications, prematurity, and low birth weight. The onset of withdrawal commonly occurs during an infant's first 2 days of life and is characterized by hyperirritability and coarse tremors, along with vomiting, diarrhea, fever, high-pitched cry, and hyperventilation; seizures and respiratory depression are less common. The production of surfactant can be accelerated in the infant of a heroin-addicted mother.

150. The answer is b. *(Behrman, 16/e, pp. 486, 497–498. McMillan, 3/e, pp. 265–266. Rudolph, 20/e, pp. 210, 226, 1593–1594.)* Idiopathic apnea is common in premature infants but is not expected in the full-term newborn. When apnea occurs, there is almost always an identifiable cause. Sepsis, gastroesophageal reflux, congenital heart disease, seizures, hypoglycemia, and airway obstruction can cause apnea in term newborns. Harlequin syndrome is a transient change in the skin color of the otherwise asymptomatic newborn (usually preterm) in which the dependent side of the entire body turns red while the upper side remains pale.

151. The answer is d. *(Behrman, 16/e, pp. 544–546, 548, 811–814. McMillan, 3/e, pp. 406–407, 858. Rudolph, 20/e, pp. 536–539.)* Neonatal sepsis, a clinical syndrome of systemic illness accompanied by bacteremia, often results in spread of infection to the meninges and other distant sites. The diagnosis of serious infection, including meningitis, in a neonate is difficult because the signs and symptoms are subtle and nonspecific. They include lethargy; feeding problems including abdominal distention, vomiting, and diarrhea; temperature instability; respiratory distress or apnea; and jaundice. Nuchal rigidity and Kernig's and Brudzinski's signs are frequently not present in the neonate with meningitis.

152. The answer is b. *(Behrman, 16/e, pp. 475–477. McMillan, 3/e, pp. 362–363. Rudolph, 20/e, pp. 243–245, 252–255.)* Twin-to-twin transfusions occur in about 15 percent of monochorionic twins and commonly cause intrauterine death. This disorder should be suspected when the hematocrits of twins differ by more than 15 mg/dL. The donor twin is likely to have oligohydramnios, anemia, and hypovolemia with evidence of shock if the hematocrit is significantly reduced; the recipient twin is likely to have hydramnios and plethora and to be larger than the donor twin. As the central venous hematocrit rises above 65 percent, infants can develop hyperviscosity, respiratory distress, hyperbilirubinemia, hypocalcemia, renal vein thrombosis, congestive heart failure, and convulsions.

153. The answer is d. *(Behrman, 16/e, pp. 32, 458, 506, 516, 1499. McMillan, 3/e, pp. 79, 165, 186–187, 192–193, 197, 262, 2224. Rudolph, 20/e, pp. 210, 225, 227, 252–255, 1134–1135, 1411–1412.)* There is loss of body weight of 1.5 percent to 2 percent per day for the first 5 days of life for a normal newborn infant as excessive fluid is excreted. This would tend to produce an increase in hematocrit, but to the contrary, the hematocrit falls as an adaptation to an environment of higher oxygen. Pulmonary artery pressure drops as the fetal cardiopulmonary system converts to air breathing. Although pulmonary arterioles are affected by pH and PCO_2 as well as by the presence of vasoactive substances, PO_2 is considered to be the major regulating influence of the pulmonary arteriolar resistance. The major smooth muscle relaxing effect of a high PO_2 causes pulmonary vascular resistance to fall. As the hematocrit falls, there is a corresponding increase in serum bilirubin. Temperature does not change.

154. The answer is c. *(Behrman, 16/e, p. 463. McMillan, 3/e, pp. 158, 309, 312, 336. Rudolph, 20/e, pp. 1055, 1069, 1350, 1867–1868.)* It is generally presumed that duodenal atresia and tracheoesophageal fistula lead to hydramnios (polyhydramnios) by interference with reabsorption of swallowed amniotic fluid. Hydramnios is also associated with approximately 80 percent of infants who have trisomy 18. Approximately 50 percent of women with anencephalic fetuses have polyhydramnios. Oligohydramnios occurs in association with congenital abnormalities of the fetal kidneys, such as renal agenesis, that inhibit formation of fetal urine.

155. The answer is e. *(Behrman, 16/e, pp. 544–546, 548–549, 981–983, 1698–1703. McMillan, 3/e, pp. 197–206, 354–355, 404–416, 429–433, 438–444, 1806–1808. Rudolph, 20/e, pp. 536–548, 610–612, 630–631, 887, 1760.)* Although hypothyroid neonates may develop hyperbilirubinemia, the patient described most likely has a congenital or acquired infection requiring immediate diagnosis and treatment. Among the important causes of neonatal sepsis are prenatal infections, including congenital syphilis, toxoplasmosis, cytomegalic inclusion disease, and rubella. Useful diagnostic studies, in addition to cultures for bacteria, include specific serologic tests for pathogens, viral cultures, lumbar puncture, and x-rays of the chest and long bones. Longitudinal striations in the metaphyses are characteristic of congenital rubella, whereas osteochondritis or periostitis usually indicates congenital syphilis. Congenital syphilis, cytomegalovirus, and rubella can be highly contagious. Urine can contain rubella virus for more than 6 months and is, therefore, a special hazard to nonimmune pregnant women.

156–159. The answers are 156–b, 157–c, 158–e, 159–a. *(Behrman, 16/e, pp. 513–517. McMillan, 3/e, pp. 197–206. Rudolph, 20/e, pp. 1133–1137.)* In premature infants who have physiologic jaundice (curve B), serum bilirubin levels rise more slowly than in term infants and usually peak at 8 to 12 mg/dL at 5 to 7 days of age; jaundice disappears after the tenth day of life. Physiologic jaundice in full-term neonates (curve D), on the other hand, usually appears at 2 to 3 days of age; peak bilirubin levels of about 5 to 6 mg/dL may appear at 2 to 4 days of age. Bilirubin levels drop below 2 mg/dL within a few days. Physiologic jaundice occurs in about one fourth to one third of all newborn infants. Jaundice usually becomes clinically apparent in these infants when the serum bilirubin exceeds about 5 to 7 mg/dL, but will depend on skin pigmentation, hematocrit, and environmental lighting. Factors contributing toward an elevation of serum levels of bilirubin in healthy neonates include the presence of an enterohepatic circulation of bilirubin, a relative increase in production of bilirubin from red-cell degradation as compared with adults, and a relative decrease in uptake, conjugation, and excretion of bilirubin by the liver. In the neonate, however, conjugation with glucuronic acid is the rate-limiting step in bilirubin metabolism that results in an increase in serum levels of unconjugated (i.e., indirect) bilirubin. Indirect bilirubin is lipid-soluble and is not expected in urine.

Jaundice in infants who have hypothyroidism (curve E) can initially appear to be physiologic. Jaundice in these infants (as well as infants who have pyloric stenosis), however, can persist for several weeks.

In neonates born with erythroblastosis fetalis (curve A), jaundice is apparent in the first 24 h of life. Bilirubin accumulates rapidly, reaching a peak level that varies with the degree of hemolysis and hepatic function. The duration of jaundice is dependent on the severity of the disease.

Curve C on the graph is compatible with a diagnosis of septicemia. In this disorder, jaundice usually appears between the fourth and seventh days of life; as the infection responds to treatment, the bilirubin levels return to normal.

160–163. The answers are 160–a, 161–c, 162–b, 163–d. (*Behrman, 16/e, pp. 470. McMillan, 3/e, pp. 155–160. Rudolph, 20/e, pp. 278–281, 336, 1602–1603.*) Tay-Sachs disease, one of the G_{M2} gangliosidoses, is diagnosed by the finding of absent or extremely low levels of leukocyte hexosaminidase A in cell samples of amniotic fluid. In heterozygous couples, levels of leukocyte hexosaminidase A are measured in chorionic villus samples taken in the first trimester of pregnancy.

An elevated level of maternal serum alpha-fetoprotein (AFP) indicates the need for further investigation. To confirm the due date and the presence of a viable singleton pregnancy, abdominal ultrasound is necessary prior to amniocentesis and may also identify a malformation responsible for the elevated AFP, such as anencephaly or other neural tube defects. A normal sonogram, however, does not eliminate the need for testing the amniotic fluid AFP levels, since serum AFP can be elevated for reasons other than neural tube defects, such as twin pregnancy, fetal death, Rh sensitization, omphalocele, congenital nephrosis, and intestinal atresia. Measurement of amniotic acetylcholinesterase, the presence of which is relatively specific for fetal neural tissue, will help to confirm the diagnosis of neural tube defect. Elevated concentrations of acetylcholinesterase in infants with ventral wall defects can be due to exposure of intestinal nerve plexuses to amniotic fluid.

Chromosomal abnormalities such as trisomy 13, 18, and 21, Turner's syndrome, and Klinefelter's syndrome can be identified prenatally by means of culture and cytogenetic examination (karyotyping) of cells derived from amniotic fluid. A low AFP (as part of the triple screen of AFP, human chorionic gonadotropin, and unconjugated estriol) can be found in Down syndrome, but the diagnosis is confirmed with chromosomes and ultrasound.

In certain clinical conditions, such as hypertensive disease of pregnancy or erythroblastosis fetalis, early delivery can be indicated. Premature delivery, however, carries a high risk of respiratory distress syndrome (RDS), a consequence of lung immaturity. Lecithin/sphingomyelin (L/S) ratio is a marker for the presence of surfaceactive phospholipids responsible for fetal lung maturation. When the L/S ratio is greater than 2:1 and the phosphatidyl glycerol is present, the risk of RDS is small; when lower than 2:1, postponement of delivery is advisable, but if postponement is not possible, the administration of glucocorticoids to accelerate lung maturation is advised for 2 to 3 days if at all feasible.

164–167. The answers are 164–a, 165–a, 166–c, 167–b. *(Behrman, 16/e, pp. 344–347, 357, 413, 1698–1703. McMillan, 3/e, pp. 354–355, 1829–1830, 1845, 1859. Rudolph, 20/e, pp. 282–288, 306–309, 313, 1142–1143, 1757–1761.)* In galactosemia, an enzyme deficiency (galactose-l-phosphate uridyl transferase) results in a block in the metabolic pathway of galactose and leads to the accumulation of galactose-l-phosphate in the tissues. Infants with this condition develop serious damage to liver, brain, and eyes after being fed milk containing lactose (a disaccharide compound of glucose and galactose). Clinical manifestations include lethargy, vomiting and diarrhea, hypotonia, hepatomegaly and jaundice, failure to thrive, and cataracts. The course of the disease in untreated patients is variable; death from liver failure and inanition can occur; most untreated patients develop physical and mental retardation. Treatment consists of prompt elimination of lactose-containing milk from the diet in infancy and, as a more varied diet is introduced, exclusion of foods that contain casein, dry milk solids, whey, or curds.

Phenylketonuria, a genetically determined disorder with an autosomal recessive pattern of inheritance, is caused by the absence of an enzyme that metabolizes phenylalanine to tyrosine. The resultant accumulation of phenylalanine and its metabolites in the blood leads to severe mental retardation in untreated patients. Treatment consists of a diet that maintains phenylalanine at levels low enough to prevent brain damage but adequate to support normal physical and mental development. Careful supervision of the low-phenylalanine diet and monitoring of blood levels are necessary. Special formulas are available for the infant; older children have difficulty following the diet. It is not clear when and if the diet can be discontinued.

Biotinidase is the enzyme responsible for breakdown of biocytin (the lysyl precursor of biotin) to free biotin. Deficiency of the enzyme, which is inherited as an autosomal recessive trait, results in malfunctioning of the biotin-dependent mitochondrial enzymes and in organic acidemia. Clinical problems related to the deficiency appear several months or years after birth and include dermatitis, alopecia, ataxia, hypotonia, seizures, developmental delay, deafness, immunodeficiency, and metabolic acidosis. The treatment is lifelong administration of free biotin.

The treatment of congenital hypothyroidism with oral levothyroxine sodium should begin as early as possible to prevent psychomotor retardation. Periodic measurement of T_3, T_4, and TSH is necessary to assess the response to therapy and the need for adjustment of the dose of thyroxine. Careful evaluation of somatic growth by plotting sequential measurements and monitoring bone age is essential.

168–171. The answers are 168–c, 169–a, 170–b, 171–b. (*Behrman, 16/e, pp. 350, 1554–1556, 1837–1838, 1901–1903, 1976, 1986. McMillan, 3/e, pp. 714–715, 727–728, 1515–1517, 2023–2025, 2251, 2255. Rudolph, 20/e, pp. 904, 946, 1284–1286, 2043–2045, 2048–2049.*) Aniridia is found in 1 percent to 2 percent of children with Wilms' tumor. Genitourinary anomalies are found in 4 percent to 5 percent and hemihypertrophy is associated with this tumor in 2 percent to 3 percent of patients.

Waardenburg's syndrome is inherited as an autosomal dominant trait with variable penetrance. It includes, in decreasing order of frequency, the following anomalies: lateral displacement of the medial canthi; broad nasal bridge; medial hyperplasia of the eyebrows; partial albinism commonly expressed by a white forelock or heterochromia (or both); and deafness in 20 percent of cases.

A flat capillary vascular malformation in the distribution of the trigeminal nerve is the basic lesion in the Sturge-Weber syndrome. The malformation also involves the meninges and results in atrophy to the underlying cerebral cortex. The damage is manifested clinically by grand mal seizures, mental deficiency, and hemiparesis or hemianopsia on the contralateral side. The cause is unknown.

Infants who have tuberous sclerosis are often born with hypopigmented oval or irregularly shaped skin macules (ash leaf). Cerebral sclerotic tubers also present from birth and become visible radiographically by the third to fourth year of life. Myoclonic seizures, present in infancy, can convert to grand mal seizures later in childhood. Adenoma sebaceum appears at 4 to 7 years of age. The disease, which also affects the eyes, kidneys, heart, bones, and lungs, is inherited as an autosomal dominant trait with variable expression; new mutations are very common.

172–174. The answers are 172–e, 173–c, 174–a. (*Behrman, 16/e, pp. 110–114, 488–489, 1189–1191, 2107. McMillan, 3/e, pp. 163, 230–235, 519–520, 610–611, 614–615. Rudolph, 20/e, pp. 213, 1877–1881, 1932, 1937, 2125.*) Subdural hematomas are commonly seen as part of the shaken baby syndrome. This lesion occurs when the bridging cortical veins that drain the cerebral cortex have been ruptured leading to a collection of blood between the dura and cerebral mantle. Repeated trauma can lead to additional collections of blood. In many children, additional findings of abuse such as broken bones, bruises, and retinal hemorrhages are found.

Caput succedaneum is soft tissue swelling of the scalp involving the presenting delivery portion of the head. This lesion is sometimes ecchymotic and can extend across the suture lines. The edema resolves in the first few days of life.

Cephalhematomas do not cross the suture line since they are subperiosteal hemorrhages. No discoloration of the scalp is seen and the swelling usually progresses over the first few hours of life. Occasionally, skull fractures are present as well. Most cephalhematomas resolve within the first few weeks or months of life without residual findings.

Intraventricular hemorrhage (IVH) is commonly seen in very small, preterm infants. The incidence of IVH increases with smaller size infants and in those with pernatal complications. It occurs in the gelatinous subependymal germinal matrix of the brain and can lead to progressive posthemorrhagic hydrocephalus. Hydrocephalus in these children can present with enlarging head circumference, apnea and bradycardia, lethargy, bulging fontanelle, widely split sutures, or no signs at all. Therapy can include ventricular-peritoneal shunting.

THE CARDIOVASCULAR SYSTEM

Questions

DIRECTIONS: Each item below contains a question or incomplete statement followed by suggested responses. Select the **one best** response to each question.

175. A 9-month-old infant accidentally ingests an unknown quantity of digitalis. The most important noncardiac manifestation of toxicity in this infant is

a. fever
b. dizziness
c. vomiting
d. visual disturbances
e. urticaria

Items 176–177

176. A 10-year-old boy complains of pain in his right knee. Two weeks ago he had a sore throat, but he did not tell anyone He is the goalie for the Salt Lake City Little League soccer team and was afraid he would miss the play-offs. Injury is a possibility, but you worry about other diagnoses. The LEAST important associated finding for confirming the suggested diagnosis is:

a. carditis
b. arthralgia
c. erythema marginatum
d. chorea
e. subcutaneous nodules

177. In the same patient, of the following manifestations of acute rheumatic fever, which is not relieved by salicylate or steroid therapy?

a. carditis
b. abdominal pain
c. arthritis
d. chorea
e. fever

178. The parents of a 2-month-old boy are concerned about his risk of coronary artery disease because of the recent death of his 40-year-old maternal uncle from a myocardial infarction. In managing this situation, you would do which of the following?

a. screen the parents for total cholesterol
b. counsel the parents regarding appropriate dietary practices for a 2-month-old infant and test him for total cholesterol at 6 months of age
c. reduce the infant's dietary fat to less than 30 percent of his calories by giving him skim milk
d. initiate lipid lowering agents
e. recommend yearly ECGs for the patient

179. For the past year, a 12-year-old boy has had recurrent episodes of swelling of his hands and feet, which has been getting worse recently. It occurs following exercise and emotional stress, lasts for 2 to 3 days, and resolves spontaneously. The last episode was accompanied by abdominal pain, vomiting, and diarrhea. The results of routine laboratory workup are normal. An older sister and a maternal uncle have had similar episodes but were not told a diagnosis. The most compatible diagnosis is

a. systemic lupus erythematosus
b. focal glomerulosclerosis
c. congenital nephrotic syndrome
d. hereditary angioedema
e. Henoch-Schönlein purpura

180. A 15-year-old girl with short stature, neck webbing, and sexual infantilism is found to have coarctation of the aorta. A chromosomal analysis would demonstrate

a. mutation at chromosome 15q21.1
b. trisomy 21
c. XO karyotype
d. defect at chromosome 4p16
e. normal chromosome analysis

181. A newborn is diagnosed with congenital heart disease. You counsel the family that the incidence of heart disease in future children is

a. 1 percent
b. 2 to 6 percent
c. 8 to 10 percent
d. 15 to 20 percent
e. 25 to 30 percent

182. During a regular checkup on an 8-year-old child, you note a loud first heart sound with a fixed and widely split second heart sound at the upper left sternal border that does not change with respirations. The patient is otherwise active and healthy. The mostly likely heart lesion to explain these findings is

a. atrial septal defect
b. ventricular septal defect
c. isolated tricuspid regurgitation
d. tetralogy of Fallot
e. mitral valve prolapse

183. A 2-year-old boy is brought into the emergency room with a complaint of fever for 6 days and development of a limp. On examination, he is found to have an erythematous macular exanthem over his body, ocular conjunctivitis, dry and cracked lips, a red throat, and cervical lymphadenopathy. There is a grade II/VI vibratory systolic ejection murmur at the lower left sternal border. A white blood cell count and differential show predominant neutrophils with increased platelets on smear. The most likely diagnosis is

a. scarlet fever
b. rheumatic fever
c. Kawasaki disease
d. juvenile rheumatoid arthritis
e. infectious mononucleosis

184. An ill-appearing 2-week-old girl is brought to the emergency room. She is pale and dyspneic with a respiratory rate of 80 breaths per min. Heart rate is 195 beats per min, heart sounds are distant, and a gallop is heard. There is cardiomegaly by x-ray. An echocardiogram demonstrates poor ventricular function, dilated ventricles, and dilation of the left atrium. An electrocardiogram shows ventricular depolarization complexes that have low voltage. The diagnosis suggested by this clinical picture is

a. myocarditis
b. endocardial fibroelastosis
c. pericarditis
d. aberrant left coronary artery arising from pulmonary artery
e. glycogen storage disease of the heart

185. A newborn infant has mild cyanosis, diaphoresis, poor peripheral pulses, hepatomegaly, and cardiomegaly. Respiratory rate is 60 breaths per min, and heart rate is 250 beats per min. The child most likely has congestive heart failure caused by

a. a large atrial septal defect and valvular pulmonic stenosis
b. a ventricular septal defect and transposition of the great vessels
c. total anomalous pulmonary venous return
d. hypoplastic left heart syndrome
e. paroxysmal atrial tachycardia

186. Congestive heart failure from congenital heart disease is encountered most frequently in which of the following age groups?

a. less than 6 months of age
b. 6 to 12 months of age
c. 1 to 5 years of age
d. 6 to 15 years of age
e. 16 to 21 years of age

187. A 2-year-old child with minimal cyanosis has a quadruple rhythm, a systolic murmur in the pulmonic area, and a mid-diastolic murmur along the lower left sternal border. An electrocardiogram shows right atrial hypertrophy and a ventricular block pattern in the right chest leads. The child most likely has

a. tricuspid regurgitation and pulmonic stenosis
b. pulmonic stenosis and a ventricular septal defect (tetralogy of Fallot)
c. an atrioventricular canal
d. Ebstein's anomaly
e. Wolff-Parkinson-White syndrome

188. A 4-year-old girl is brought to the pediatrician's office. Her father reports that she suddenly became pale and stopped running while he had been playfully chasing her. After 30 min, she was no longer pale and wanted to resume the game. She has never had a previous episode or ever been cyanotic. Her physical examination was normal as were her chest x-ray and echocardiogram. An electrocardiogram showed the pattern seen in the following figure, which indicates

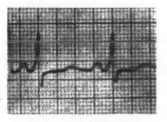

a. paroxysmal ventricular tachycardia
b. paroxysmal supraventricular tachycardia
c. Wolff-Parkinson-White syndrome
d. Stokes-Adams pattern
e. excessive stress during play

189. A child has a history of spiking fevers, which have been as high as 40°C (104°F). She has spindle-shaped swelling of finger joints and complains of upper sternal pain. The most likely diagnosis is

a. rheumatic fever
b. juvenile rheumatoid arthritis
c. toxic synovitis
d. septic arthritis
e. osteoarthritis

190. A cyanotic newborn is suspected of having congenital heart disease. The ECG shows left axis deviation and left ventricular hypertrophy (LVH). The most likely diagnosis is

a. transposition of the great arteries
b. truncus arteriosus
c. tricuspid atresia
d. tetralogy of Fallot
e. persistent fetal circulation

191. A 3-day-old infant with a single second heart sound has had progressively deepening cyanosis since birth but no respiratory distress. Chest radiography demonstrates no cardiomegaly and normal pulmonary vasculature. An electrocardiogram shows an axis of 120 degrees and right ventricular prominence. The congenital cardiac malformation most likely responsible for the cyanosis is

a.   tetralogy of Fallot
b.   transposition of the great vessels
c.   tricuspid atresia
d.   pulmonary atresia with intact ventricular septum
e.   total anomalous pulmonary venous return below the diaphragm

192. During a physical examination for participation in a sport, a 16-year-old girl is noted to have a late apical systolic murmur, which is preceded by a click. The rest of the cardiac examination is normal. She states that her mother also has some type of heart "murmur" but knows nothing else about it. The most likely diagnosis is

a.   atrial septal defect
b.   aortic stenosis
c.   tricuspid regurgitation
d.   mitral valve prolapse
e.   ventricular septal defect

193. Appropriate management for the patient in the previous question includes

a.   cardiac catheterization
b.   penicillin prophylaxis for dental procedures
c.   avoidance of strenuous activity
d.   beta blockers (propanolol)
e.   digitalis

DIRECTIONS: Each group of questions below consists of lettered options followed by numbered items. For each numbered item, select the appropriate lettered option(s). Each lettered option may be used once, more than once, or not at all. **Choose exactly the number of options indicated following each item.**

Items 194–196

For each major cardiovascular abnormality listed below, select the syndrome with which it is most likely to be associated.

a. Holt-Oram syndrome
b. Turner's syndrome
c. Marfan's syndrome
d. Williams syndrome
e. Down syndrome

194. Coarctation of the aorta
(SELECT 1 SYNDROME)

195. Endocardial cushion defect
(SELECT 1 SYNDROME)

196. Aortic aneurysm
(SELECT 1 SYNDROME)

Items 197–200

For each condition, select the most appropriate treatment.

a. packed red blood cells
b. Ringer's lactate
c. whole blood
d. 5% dextrose in water contain ing 40 mEq/L of sodium chloride and 20 mEq/L of potassium acetate
e. 10% dextrose in water without electrolytes

197. Severe anemia
(SELECT 1 TREATMENT)

198. Continuing massive bleeding in a patient in shock
(SELECT 1 TREATMENT)

199. Prevention of dehydration in a patient who is receiving nothing by mouth prior to surgery
(SELECT 1 TREATMENT)

200. Circulatory collapse in a dehydrated infant
(SELECT 1 TREATMENT)

THE CARDIOVASCULAR SYSTEM

Answers

175. The answer is c. *(Behrman, 16/e, pp. 2254. Rudolph, 20/e, pp. 1537–1539.)* An important noncardiac manifestation of digitalis toxicity in infants is vomiting. Affected infants also exhibit electrocardiographic changes, including sinus arrhythmia (bradycardia) and a wandering pacemaker, paroxysmal tachycardia, and a heart rate of less than 100 beats per min. The commonly used digitalis preparation in infants is digoxin. Digoxin blood levels of 2 ng/dL or less are usually therapeutic in adults; in contrast, therapeutic digoxin blood levels in infants range from 1 to 5 ng/dL, but the benefit of the higher levels in infants is doubtful.

176–177. The answers are 176–b, 177–d. *(Behrman, 16/e, pp. 806–810. McMillan, 3/e, pp. 1417–1422. Rudolph, 20/e, pp. 1518–1521.)* It is often difficult to establish a diagnosis of rheumatic fever because there is no single clinical manifestation or laboratory test that is confirmatory. The importance of doing so relates to the need to treat the acute problems promptly and effectively as well as to the importance of instituting long-term antibiotic prophylaxis to prevent recurrences. To assist in diagnosis, the American Heart Association identified a set of major and minor standards relating to the manifestations of the disease called the Jones criteria (modified) and recommends that these criteria be applied in the diagnosis of every patient with possible rheumatic fever. The major criteria are carditis, arthritis, erythema marginatum, chorea, and subcutaneous nodules. The minor criteria are arthralgia (joint pain with no objective findings), fever or history of rheumatic fever, increased erythrocyte sedimentation rate (ESR), positive C-reactive protein, increased WBC and anemia, and prolonged PR and QT intervals on ECG. To make the diagnosis of rheumatic fever, the following criteria should be met: two major manifestations, or one major and two minors plus strong evidence of a preceding group A β-hemolytic streptococcal infection (culture, rapid antigen-antibody rise or elevation) or scarlet fever.

Administration of salicylates and steroids can relieve the inflammatory manifestations of acute rheumatic fever. Steroids are used to treat affected children who have carditis with an enlarged heart. Neither salicylates nor corticosteroids have a therapeutic effect on chorea, but barbiturates and chlorpromazine may be helpful.

178. The answer is a. (*Behrman, 16/e, pp. 389–390. McMillan, 3/e, pp. 1864–1865. Rudolph, 20/e, pp. 345–347.*) Identification of those with a genetic predisposition to hypercholesterolemia and of the factors that increase the risk of the condition is recommended so that dietary and other measures to reduce serum lipids can be introduced if indicated. Children with a first- or second-degree relative with early onset of coronary heart disease should be evaluated early in life but after 2 years of age. Other known risk factors include obesity, diabetes, hypertension, and smoking. No change in current infant dietary practice is recommended for children under 2 years of age. The high total fat content of the infant diet is considered to be biologically sound given the need for lipid for a developing nervous system and the infant's limited capacity for an intake of high volume during this period of rapid growth. It is generally agreed that a dietary fat intake ≥ 40 percent of calories is excessive over the age of 2 years. There is, however, concern about the potential loss of minerals such as iron, zinc, and calcium when dietary fat is reduced below 30 percent of calories in children 2 to 18 years of age. Principal sources of fat in the American diet are meat and milk, which are also sources of minerals such as iron and calcium. Simple modifications in the current U.S. diet of children of these ages (trimming excess fat from meat and drinking 1% fat milk) would effect a reduction of fat intake by 5 percent of calories without the risk of lowering mineral intake. It would be helpful in this situation to determine whether the uncle had hypercholesterolemia. Yearly ECGs and lipid lowering agents are not indicated in this situation.

179. The answer is d. (*Behrman, 16/e, pp. 632–633, 684–685. McMillan, 3/e, pp. 2051–2052. Rudolph, 20/e, pp. 451, 473–474.*) This condition often worsens in adolescents. Although hereditary angioedema is relatively rare as a cause of edema, the recurrent episodes in late childhood, the normal laboratory results, and the family history make the other choices less likely. Hereditary angioedema, transmitted as an autosomal dominant trait, is due to inadequate function (due to either deficient quantity or quality) of an inhibitor of the first step in the complement cascade, which results in the excessive production of a vasoactive kinin. In addition to otherwise asymptomatic subcutaneous edema, edema can occur in the gastrointestinal tract and produce the symptoms mentioned in the question. Laryngeal edema with airway obstruction can also occur.

180. The answer is c. *(Behrman, 16/e, pp. 330, 1753–1755. McMillan, 3/e, pp. 1352, 1893–1895, 2142, 2230–2231. Rudolph, 20/e, pp. 298, 383, 392–393, 1782–1784, 1978.)* Short stature, neck webbing, sexual infantilism, and a shieldlike chest with widely spaced nipples are signs of Turner's syndrome, which is usually associated with an XO karyotype. Aortic coarctation occurs in about 15 percent to 20 percent of those with this disorder. Down syndrome is most commonly associated with endocardial cushing defects or ventricular septal defect. Marfan's syndrome (mutation 15q21.1) is associated with dilatation of the aorta and mitral and aortic regurgitation. Ellis-van Creveld syndrome (defect is 4p16) is associated with atrial septal defects.

181. The answer is b. *(Behrman, 16/e, p. 1363. McMillan, 3/e, p. 279. Rudolph, 20/e, pp. 1457–1458.)* The incidence of congenital heart disease in the population is about 1 percent. The risk of congenital heart disease in a family with one child born with heart disease varies depending on the type of lesion the first child had but, overall, the rate averages from about 2 percent to 6 percent if the heart disease is not associated with a diagnosable syndrome. The risk of congenital heart disease for an infant is increased if there is a history of congenital heart disease in the mother. If there are two children with congenital heart disease, the risk escalates to 20 percent to 30 percent.

182. The answer is a. *(Behrman, 16/e, pp. 1365–1366, 1369–1371, 1383–1390. McMillan, 3/e, pp. 287, 1329–1332, 1346–1350, 1354–1357, 1378–1380. Rudolph, 20/e, pp. 1466–1469, 1474–1475, 1497–1502.)* Most commonly, children with an atrial septal defect (ASD) are asymptomatic with the lesion found during a routine examination. In older children, exercise intolerance can be noted if the lesion is of significant size. On examination, the pulses are normal, a right ventricular systolic lift at the left sternal border is palpable, and a fixed splitting of the second heart sound is audible. For lesser degrees of ASD, surgical treatment is more controversial. Ventricular septal defects commonly present as a harsh or blowing holosystolic murmur best heard along the left lower sternum, often with radiation throughout the precordium. Tricuspid regurgitation is a mid-diastolic rumble at the lower left sternal border. Often, a history of birth asphyxia or findings of other cardiac lesions are present. Tetralogy of Fallot is a very common form of congenital heart disease. The four abnormalities include right ventricular outflow obstruction, ventricular septal defect, dextroposition of the aorta, and right ventricular hypertrophy. The cyanosis presents in infants and in young children. Mitral valve prolapse occurs with the billowing into the atria of one or both mitral valve leaflets at the end of systole. It is a congenital abnormality that frequently only manifests during adolescence or later. It is more common in girls than in boys and seems to be inherited in an autosomal dominant fashion. On clinical examination, an apical murmur is noted late in systole, which can be preceded by a mid systolic click. The diagnosis is confirmed with an echocardiogram that shows prolapse of the mitral leaflets during mid to late systole. Antibiotic prophylaxis is recommended for dental work (especially if a murmur is present) as the incidence of endocarditis can be higher in these patients.

183. The answer is c. (*Behrman, 16/e, pp. 725–727. McMillan, 3/e, pp. 924–932. Rudolph, 20/e, pp. 495–497.*) Many conditions can be associated with prolonged fever, a limp caused by arthralgia, exanthem, adenopathy, and pharyngitis. Conjunctivitis, however, is suggestive of Kawasaki disease. The fissured lips, although common in Kawasaki disease, could occur after a long period of fever from any cause if the child became dehydrated. The predominance of neutrophils and high sedimentation rate are common to all. An increase in platelets within this constellation of symptoms, however, is found only in Kawasaki disease. Kawasaki disease presents a picture of prolonged fever, rash, epidermal peeling on the hands and feet (especially around the fingertips), conjunctivitis, lymphadenopathy, fissured lips, oropharyngeal mucosal erythema, and arthralgia or arthritis. The diagnosis is still possible in the absence of one or two of these physical findings. Coronary artery aneurysms can develop.

184. The answer is a. (*Behrman, 16/e, pp. 1434–1435. McMillan, 3/e, pp. 1389–1397. Rudolph, 20/e, pp. 1326–1330.*) The findings of pallor, dyspnea, tachypnea, tachycardia, and cardiomegaly are common in congestive heart failure regardless of the cause. The most common causes of myocarditis include adenovirus and Coxsackievirus B, although many other viruses can cause this condition. The constellation of findings in the question point to myocarditis as the etiology of this patient's condition. The lack of echocardiographic findings other than ventricular and left atrial dilatation and poor ventricular function is inconsistent with both glycogen storage disease of the heart, in which there is muscle thickening, and pericarditis, since there is no pericardial effusion. It is also not consistent with an aberrant origin of the left coronary artery although the origin of the coronary arteries can be more easily missed. On electrocardiogram, the voltages of the ventricular complexes seen with aberrant origin of the left coronary artery are not diminished and a pattern of myocardial infarction can be seen. Voltages from the left ventricle are usually high in endocardial fibroelastosis, and both right and left ventricular forces are high in glycogen storage disease of the heart.

185. The answer is e. *(Behrman, 16/e, pp. 1418–1421. McMillan, 3/e, pp. 290–291, 1431–1432. Rudolph, 20/e, pp. 1452–1453.)* Congestive heart failure from any cause can result in mild cyanosis, even in the absence of a right-to-left shunt, and in poor peripheral pulses when cardiac output is low. Congestive heart failure from many causes can be associated with a rapid pulse rate (up to 200 beats per min). A pulse rate greater than 250 beats per min, however, should suggest the presence of a tachyarrhythmia. Common causes for supraventricular tachycardia includes Wolff-Parkinson-White (WPW) syndrome, congenital heart disease, and sympathomimetic drugs. In this patient, evaluation for WPW and cardiac abnormalities must be accomplished after the congestive heart failure from the increased heart rate is under control.

186. The answer is a. *(Behrman, 16/e, pp. 1440–1444. McMillan, 3/e, p. 298. Rudolph, 20/e, pp. 1533–1536.)* The greatest cause of congestive heart failure in children is congenital heart disease. Congestive heart failure from congenital heart disease most often occurs in infants during their first weeks of life. Other causes of heart failure in young infants include primary myocardial disease, metabolic abnormalities, anemia, and paroxysmal atrial tachycardia; other causes, such as bacterial endocarditis and rheumatic heart disease, are rare in the first year of life.

187. The answer is d. *(Behrman, 16/e, pp. 1384, 1393–1395. Rudolph, 20/e, pp. 1505–1506.)* A quadruple rhythm associated with the murmur of tricuspid regurgitation and a mid-diastolic murmur at the lower left sternum suggests the diagnosis of Ebstein's anomaly (downward displacement of the tricuspid valve). The presence of right atrial hypertrophy and right ventricular conduction defects confirms the diagnosis. Both tricuspid regurgitation with pulmonic stenosis and tetralogy of Fallot give electrocardiographic evidence of right ventricular enlargement. The Wolff-Parkinson-White syndrome, which frequently accompanies Ebstein's malformation, is not associated with murmurs or cyanosis as an isolated entity but also includes supraventricular tachycardia.

188. The answer is c. *(Behrman, 16/e, pp. 1418–1420. McMillan, 3/e, pp. 1431–1432. Rudolph, 20/e, pp. 1452–1453.)* The child described in the question, who has no cyanosis or murmur, no cardiac or pulmonary vascular abnormalities by chest x-ray, and no evidence of structural anomalies by echocardiogram, is unlikely to have an underlying gross anatomic defect. The electrocardiographic pattern in the figure shows the configuration of preexcitation, the pattern seen in the Wolff-Parkinson-White syndrome (WPW). These patients have an aberrant atrioventricular conduction pathway, which causes the early ventricular depolarization appearing on the electrocardiogram as a shortened PR interval. The initial slow ventricular depolarization wave is referred to as the delta wave. Seventy percent of patients with WPW have single or repeated episodes of paroxysmal supraventricular tachycardia, which can cause the symptoms described in the question. The preexcitation electrocardiographic pattern and WPW can occur in Ebstein's malformation, but this is unlikely in the absence of cyanosis and with a normal echocardiogram. If ventricular tachycardia were present, the symptoms would likely be more profound. Active play and exposure to over-the-counter medications containing sympathomimetics in a healthy 4-year-old child can cause symptoms such as those described in the question in children with WPW by precipitating paroxysmal supraventricular tachycardia.

189. The answer is b. *(Behrman, 16/e, pp. 704–709. McMillan, 3/e, pp. 2156–2160. Rudolph, 20/e, pp. 479–483.)* Juvenile rheumatoid arthritis (JRA) frequently causes spindle-shaped swelling of finger joints and can involve unusual joints such as the sternoclavicular joint. Presentation of

JRA occurs as either polyarthritis (5 or more joints, systemic symptoms not so severe or persistent), pauciarticular (4 or few joints, lower extremity joints, extra articular disease unusual), or systemic disease (severe constitutional disease, systemic symptoms prior to arthritis, rheumatoid rash, high spiking fevers, variable joints). This disorder can be associated with spiking high fevers, which are not a feature of rheumatic fever, toxic synovitis, or osteoarthritis. Although septic arthritis can affect any joint, it would not be likely to affect finger joints by causing spindle-shaped swellings. Toxic synovitis usually involves larger joints such as the hip, and osteoarthritis is not a disease of childhood.

190. The answer is c. *(Behrman, 16/e, pp. 1391–1392. McMillan, 3/e, pp. 1327–1329. Rudolph, 20/e, pp. 1502–1503.)* Tricuspid atresia has a hypoplastic right ventricle and, therefore, the ECG shows left axis deviation and left ventricular hypertrophy. Almost all other forms of cyanotic congenital heart disease are associated with elevated pressures in the right ventricle. In those, therefore, the ECG will show right axis deviation and right ventricular hypertrophy.

191. The answer is b. *(Behrman, 16/e, pp. 1395–1398. McMillan, 3/e, pp. 1322–1324. Rudolph, 20/e, pp. 1506–1509.)* Transposition of the great vessels with an intact ventricular septum presents with early cyanosis, a normal-sized heart (classic "egg on a string" radiographic pattern in one third of cases), normal or slightly increased pulmonary vascular markings, and an electrocardiogram showing right axis deviation and right ventricular hypertrophy. In tetralogy of Fallot, cyanosis is often not seen in the first few days of life. Tricuspid atresia, a cause of early cyanosis, causes diminished pulmonary arterial blood flow; the pulmonary fields on x-ray demonstrate a diminution of pulmonary vascularity. There is a left axis and left ventricular hypertrophy shown by electrocardiogram. Total anomalous pulmonary venous return below the diaphragm is associated with obstruction to pulmonary venous return and a classic radiographic finding of marked, fluffy-appearing venous congestion ("snowman"). In pulmonic atresia with intact ventricular septum, cyanosis appears early, the lung markings are normal to diminished, and the heart is large.

192–193. The answers are 192–d, 193–b. *(Behrman, 16/e, pp. 1383–1384. McMillan, 3/e, pp. 1378–1380.)* Mitral valve prolapse occurs with the billowing into the atria of one or both mitral valve leaflets at the end of systole. It is a congenital abnormality that frequently only manifests during adolescence or later. It is more common in girls than in boys and seems to be inherited in an autosomal dominant fashion. On clinical examination, an apical murmur is noted late in systole, which can be preceded by a click. The diagnosis is confirmed with an echocardiogram that shows prolapse of the mitral leaflets during mid to late systole. The ECG and chest x-ray are usually normal. Beta blockers and digitalis are unlikely to be required, but penicillin prophylaxis for dental procedures for patients with mitral valve prolapse, especially if a murmur is present, is indicated.

194–196. The answers are 194–b, 195–e, 196–c. *(Behrman, 16/e, pp. 328, 331, 1365–1366, 1377, 1753–1755, 2131–2132. McMillan, 3/e, pp. 1347, 2230–2231, 2241, 2251. Rudolph, 20/e, pp. 297 299, 392–394, 1782–1784.)* Common features of Turner's syndrome include female phenotype, short stature, sexual infantilism, streak gonads, broad chest, low hairline, webbed neck, congenital lymphedema of the hands and feet, coarctation of the aorta, and a variety of other anomalies.

Down syndrome has many diagnostic features including microcephaly, centrally placed hair whorl, small ears, redundant skin on the nape of the neck, upslanting palpebral fissures, epicanthal folds, flat nasal bridge, Brushfield's spots, protruding tongue, short and broad hands, simian creases, widely spaced first and second toe, and hypotonia. Cardiac lesions are found in 30 percent to 50 percent of children with Down syndrome, including endocardial cushion defect (30 percent), ventricular septal defect (30 percent), and tetralogy of Fallot (about 30 percent).

Major findings in Marfan's syndrome include ectopia lentis (subluxation of the ocular lens), progressive dilatation of the aortic root and ascending aorta, aortic aneurysm, excessive height for age, and disproportionately long and thin extremities.

Holt-Oram syndrome includes an atrial septal defect with skeletal abnormalities primarily of the forearm and hand. Williams syndrome is most characteristically associated with supraventricular aortic stenosis, peripheral pulmonic stenosis, pulmonary valve stenosis, atrial septal defect, and ventricular septal defect.

197–200. The answers are 197–a, 198–c, 199–d, 200–b. *(Behrman, 16/e, pp. 215–216, 220, 262–266, 1499–1500. McMillan, 3/e, pp. 70, 363,*

1457–1459, 2194–2195, 2212. Rudolph, 20/e, pp. 1186–1188, 1252–1253, 1325–1326.) With severe chronic anemia, plasma volume will already be expanded and it is, therefore, important to increase red-cell volume with a minimal increase in blood volume. This can be done by a partial exchange transfusion or by the slow infusion of packed red blood cells, which allows time for physiologic mechanisms involving the liver and kidney to reduce plasma volume.

A patient in shock with continuing bleeding needs replacement of blood volume, and this can be done best with whole blood or by administering both packed cells and plasma.

To prevent dehydration, a solution containing some glucose and small amounts of sodium, potassium, and basic anions will provide all that is needed for a few days. The other products would, therefore, be unnecessary and add the dangers associated with transfusion of blood and blood products.

With circulatory shock in a dehydrated infant, it is important to rapidly expand blood volume so that tissue perfusion improves and renal and cardiopulmonary systems can function to correct the disturbances that have been produced. Of the solutions given, the Ringer's lactate would be best, but if the patient was also anemic, then whole blood or packed cells could also be used if it could be made available quickly enough. Solution d. would not be appropriate, since it is too low in sodium to expand extracellular volume adequately. A solution with a higher sodium concentration in the range of 90 to 150 mEq/L, however, could be used (normal saline).

THE RESPIRATORY SYSTEM

Questions

DIRECTIONS: Each item below contains a question or incomplete statement followed by suggested responses. Select the **one best** response to each question.

Items 201–202

201. A previously well 1-year-old infant has had a runny nose and has been sneezing and coughing for 2 days. Two other members of the family had similar symptoms. Four hours ago, his cough became much worse. On physical examination, he is in moderate respiratory distress with nasal flaring, hyperexpansion of the chest, and easily audible wheezing without rales. The most likely diagnosis is

a.   bronchiolitis
b.   viral croup
c.   asthma
d.   epiglottitis
e.   diphtheria

202. The most likely agent responsible for the infant's condition in the previous question is

a.   *Staphylococcus aureus*
b.   *Haemophilus influenzae*
c.   *Corynebacterium diphtheriae*
d.   respiratory syncytial virus
e.   ECHO virus

203. A 10-month-old infant has poor weight gain, a persistent cough, and a history of several bouts of pneumonitis. The mother describes the child as having very large, foul-smelling stools for months. Which of the following diagnostic maneuvers is likely to result in the diagnosis of this child?

a.   CT of the chest
b.   serum immunoglobulins
c.   TB skin test
d.   inspiratory and expiratory chest x-ray
e.   sweat chloride test

204. A 13-year-old girl with a history of 2 days of cough and fever has the chest x-ray shown in the following figure. The most appropriate treatment is

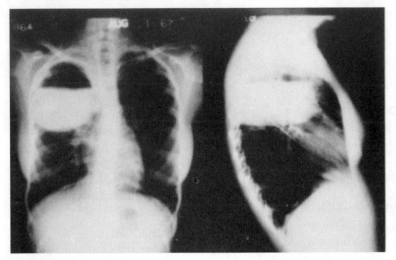

a.   N-acetylcysteine
b.   prolonged course of ampicillin combined with a beta lactamase inhibitor
c.   lobectomy
d.   postural drainage
e.   thoracentesis and chest tube

205. Which of the following ingested agents is most likely to produce respiratory symptoms?

a.   motor oil
b.   castor oil
c.   oil of wintergreen
d.   furniture polish
e.   mineral oil

206. A 3-year-old girl is admitted with the x-ray pictured. The child lives with her parents and a 6-week-old brother. Her grandfather stayed with the family for 2 months before his return to the West Indies 1 month ago. The grandfather had a 3-month history of weight loss, fever, and hemoptysis. Appropriate management of this problem includes

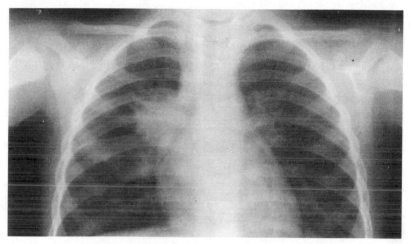

(Courtesy Susan John, M.D.)

a. bronchoscopy and culture of washings for all family members
b. placement of a Mantoux test on the 6-week-old sibling
c. isolating the 3-year-old patient for 1 month
d. treating the 3-year-old patient with INH and rifampin
e. HIV testing for all family members

207. A tine test administered at a routine visit of a 2½-year-old boy is positive. The child is asymptomatic and thriving; there is no known exposure to tuberculosis. Your initial course of action would be to

a. admit the child and perform a workup for tuberculosis
b. start the child on isoniazid
c. repeat the tine test
d. screen all contacts with a tuberculin test and chest x-ray
e. administer a Mantoux (PPD) test

208. A previously healthy, active 18-month-old child presents with unilateral nasal obstruction and foul-smelling discharge. The child's examination is otherwise unremarkable. The most likely diagnosis is

a. foreign body
b. nasal polyps
c. frontal sinusitis
d. deviated septum
e. choanal atresia

209. Which of the following therapies is to be avoided in a child with obstructive sleep apnea?

a. insertion of an airway
b. nasal continuous positive airway pressure (CPAP)
c. tonsillectomy and adenoidectomy
d. irradiation of the tonsillar bed
e. a trial of steroids

210. A patient with staphylococcal pneumonia suddenly develops increasing respiratory distress. The possible diagnosis requiring the most urgent action is

a. pneumatocele formation
b. tension pneumothorax
c. progression of the pneumonia
d. severe anxiety
e. pleural effusion

211. Which of the following is an absolute indication for tonsillectomy?

a. repeated ear infections
b. three throat infections in the previous year
c. mouth breathing
d. frequent upper respiratory infections
e. need to rule out tumor

212. A 6-year-old boy is brought to the emergency room with a 3-h history of fever to 39.5°C (103.1°F) and sore throat. The child appears alert but anxious and he has mild inspiratory stridor. You should immediately

a. examine the throat and obtain a culture
b. obtain an arterial blood gas and start an IV line
c. order a chest x-ray and lateral view of the neck
d. prepare to establish an airway
e. admit the child and place him in a mist tent

213. A 3-year-old boy has a young puppy and a history of pica. He has a recent onset of wheezing, hepatomegaly, and marked eosinophilia (80 percent eosinophils). The test most likely to produce a specific diagnosis is

a. tuberculin skin test
b. histoplasmin test
c. ELISA for *Toxocara*
d. silver stain of gastric aspirate
e. stool examination for ova and parasites

214. A 10-year-old has had a "cold" for 14 days. In the 2 days prior to the visit to your office, she has developed a fever to 39°C (102.2°F), purulent nasal discharge, facial pain, and a daytime cough. Examination of the nose after topical decongestants shows pus in the middle meatus. The most likely diagnosis is

a. brain abscess
b. maxillary sinusitis
c. streptococcal throat infection
d. frontal sinusitis
e. middle ear infection

215. You are awakened in the night by your 2-year-old son, who has developed noisy breathing on inspiration, marked retractions of the chest wall, flaring of the nostrils, and a barking cough. He has had a mild upper respiratory infection (URI) for 2 days. The most likely diagnosis is

a. asthma
b. epiglottitis
c. bronchiolitis
d. viral croup
e. foreign body in the right mainstem bronchus

216. In patients on theophylline therapy for asthma, certain other drugs change theophylline clearance and raise or lower theophylline levels. Which of the following medications may be safely administered with theophylline?

a. erythromycin
b. phenytoin
c. cimetidine
d. rifampin
e. penicillin

217. A 13-year-old develops fever, malaise, sore throat, and a dry hacking cough over several days. He does not appear to be particularly sick, but his chest examination is significant for diffuse rales and rhonchi. Chest x-ray shows peribronchial thickening and some subsegmental atelectasis. The most likely pathogen is

a. *Staphylococcus aureus*
b. *Mycobacterium tuberculosis*
c. *Haemophilus influenzae*
d. *Streptococcus pneumoniae*
e. *Mycoplasma pneumoniae*

218. As a doctor in a clinic, you have just given a 10-year-old boy an injection of pollen extract as prescribed by his allergist. You are about to move on to the next patient when the boy starts to complain about a funny feeling in his chest, and his face becomes red and swollen. He then develops severe respiratory distress with wheezing, and as he starts to fall, you catch him and place him on a bed. The LEAST important measure to be instituted immediately would be

a. endotracheal intubation
b. placement of a tourniquet above the injection site
c. administration of oxygen
d. subcutaneous injection of 1:1000 epinephrine 0.2 mL
e. administration of corticosteroids

219. A previously healthy 18-month-old has been in a separate room from his family. The family notices the sudden onset of coughing, which resolves over a few minutes. Subsequently, the patient appears to be normal except for increased amounts of drooling and refusal to take foods orally. The most likely explanation for this toddler's condition is

a. severe gastroesophageal reflux
b. foreign body in the airway
c. croup
d. epiglottitis
e. foreign body in the esophagus

Items 220–223

220. You receive a telephone call from the mother of a 4-year-old child with sickle cell anemia. She tells you that the child is breathing fast, coughing, and has a temperature of 104°F (40°C). The most conservative, prudent approach is to

a. prescribe aspirin and ask her to call back if the fever does not respond
b. make an office appointment for the next available opening
c. make an office appointment for the next day
d. refer the child to the laboratory for an immediate hematocrit, white blood cell count, and differential
e. admit the child to the hospital as an emergency

221. Although the patient is in respiratory distress, a lack of cyanosis indicates

a. insignificant hypoxia
b. that the patient has pulmonary thrombi rather than pneumonia
c. very little since it is not a useful indication of hypoxia in a patient with anemia
d. shift of the oxyhemoglobin curve to the right due to increased levels of BPG (previously known as DPG)
e. an adequate hemoglobin level for the given activity level

222. The laboratory workup of the patient reveals the following: hemoglobin 5 g/dL; hematocrit 16; white blood cell count 30,000/mm^3; and arterial blood, while breathing room air, of pH 7.1, Po$_2$ 5 mmHg, and Pco$_2$ 8 mm Hg. These values indicate

a. acidemia, metabolic acidosis, respiratory alkalosis, and hypoxia
b. alkalemia, respiratory acidosis, metabolic alkalosis, and hypoxia
c. acidosis with compensatory hypoventilation
d. long-term metabolic compensation for respiratory alkalosis
e. primary respiratory alkalosis

223. While waiting for further studies of the patient, it is appropriate to administer

a. sedation
b. bicarbonate by IV push
c. urea
d. 100% oxygen
e. 40% oxygen with 5% carbon dioxide

224. A 13-year-old boy has a 3-day history of low-grade fever, upper respiratory symptoms, and a sore throat. A few hours before his presentation to the emergency room, he has an abrupt onset of high fevers, difficulty swallowing, and poor handling of his secretions. He indicates that he has a marked worsening in the severity of his sore throat. His pharynx has a fluctuant bulge in the posterior wall. Appropriate initial therapy for this patient would be

a. narcotic analgesics
b. trial of oral penicillin V
c. surgical consultation for incision and drainage under general anesthesia
d. rapid streptococcal screen
e. monospot test

225. A 6-week-old child develops increased respiratory rate and a non-productive cough. Physical examination is significant for rales and rhonchi. The past medical history for the child is positive for an eye discharge at 3 weeks of age, which was treated with a topical antibiotic drug. The most likely organism causing this child's condition is

a. *Neisseria gonorrhoeae*
b. *Staphylococcus aureus*
c. Group B streptococcus
d. *Chlamydia trachomatis*
e. herpes virus

226. Appropriate therapy for the patient in the previous question includes

a. ceftriaxone
b. acyclovir
c. penicillin G
d. nafcillin
e. erythromycin

227. A previously healthy 2-year-old black child has developed a chronic cough over the previous 6 weeks. He has been seen in different emergency rooms on two occasions during this period and placed on antibiotics for pneumonia. Upon auscultation, you hear normal breath sounds on the left. On the right side, you hear decreased air movement during inspiration but none upon expiration. The routine chest radiograph shows no infiltrate, but the heart is shifted slightly to the left. The appropriate next step in making the diagnosis in this patient is to

a. measure the patient's sweat chloride
b. obtain inspiratory and expiratory chest radiographs
c. prescribe broad-spectrum oral antibiotics
d. initiate a trial of inhaled beta-agonists
e. prescribe appropriate doses of oral prednisone

DIRECTIONS: Each group of questions below consists of lettered options followed by numbered items. For each numbered item, select the appropriate lettered option(s). Each lettered option may be used once, more than once, or not at all. **Choose exactly the number of options indicated following each item.**

Items 228–230

Match each management procedure below with the appropriate set of arterial blood gas results of patients spontaneously breathing room air.

	pH	P_{CO_2} (mm Hg)	P_{O_2} (mm Hg)	Base Excess (mEq/L)
(A)	7.20	28	95	216
(B)	7.20	70	41	22
(C)	7.64	18	94	21
(D)	7.34	32	39	28
(E)	none of the above			

228. Have patient rebreathe in a paper bag   C

229. Administer F_{IO_2} 0.4

230. Perform thoracentesis to remove air under pressure

Items 231–234

Match each management procedure below with the appropriate arterial blood gas results of patients spontaneously breathing room air.

	pH	P_{CO_2} (mm Hg)	P_{O_2} (mm Hg)	Base Excess (mEq/L)
(A)	6.92	101	19	215
(B)	7.36	60	50	17
(C)	7.50	46	76	111
(D)	7.41	60	90	110
(E)	none of the above			

231. Place the patient on a ventilator with an F_{IO_2} of 1.0

232. Discontinue diuretics, discontinue base, and increase KCl in IV fluids

233. Perform tonsillectomy

234. Repeat the test because of obvious laboratory error

THE RESPIRATORY SYSTEM

Answers

201–202. The answers are 201-a, 202-d. *(Behrman, 16/e, pp. 1285–1287. McMillan, 3/e, pp. 1214–1216. Rudolph, 20/e, pp. 672–677.)* Of the choices given, bronchiolitis is the most likely, although asthma, pertussis, and bronchopneumonia can present similarly. The family history of upper respiratory infections, the previous upper respiratory illness in the patient, and signs of intrathoracic airway obstruction make the diagnosis of bronchiolitis more likely. Viral croup, epiglottitis, and diphtheria are not reasonable choices because there are no signs of extrathoracic airway obstruction.

The most likely cause of the illness is infection by respiratory syncytial virus, which causes outbreaks of bronchiolitis of varying severity, usually in the winter and spring. Other viruses, such as parainfluenza and the adenoviruses, have also been implicated in producing bronchiolitis. Treatment is usually supportive in this usually self-limited condition. Ribavirin, an expensive antiviral agent, is reserved for the most severe cases, those who have congenital heart disease, BPD, immune deficiency, and chest wall abnormalities.

203. The answer is e. *(Behrman, 16/e, pp. 1315–1327. McMillan, 3/e, pp. 1242–1254. Rudolph, 20/e, 1640–1650.)* Cystic fibrosis (CF) is a multisystem disease caused by an abnormally functioning cystic fibrosis transmembrane regulator protein. Abnormal secretions are produced as a result of decreased permeability of ionized chloride in the secretory epithelium of a number of organs. Progressive lung failure is caused by accumulation of viscid secretions that obstruct the airway and lead to infection, bronchiectasis, and inflammatory changes. Survival has improved during the past few decades as a result of prompt recognition of CF and aggressive treatment; the median age at death has increased from less than 10 years to more than 30 years. Therapeutic approaches have included inhalation therapy, chest physical therapy, aggressive antibiotic administration, bronchodilators, oxygen, and nutritional support. Heart–lung transplants have prolonged life and improved quality of life for some terminal patients. Several new approaches to the treatment of CF have been proposed, namely, the use of amiloride, purified human plasma $alpha_1$-antitrypsin, recombinant DNAase, and gene therapy. The rationale for these therapeutic modalities is that they focus directly on ameliorating or correcting the basic deficit: amiloride by inhibiting sodium, and with it water reabsorption, and thereby improving airway hydration; $alpha_1$-antitrypsin by counteracting the effects on the lungs of neutrophil elastase, a proteolytic enzyme released by neutrophils; DNAase by reacting with DNA released by dead leukocytes to reduce sputum viscosity; and gene therapy by altering genetic material. Lung cancer does not appear to be associated with cystic fibrosis.

Unlike many other tests, there is almost no overlap in chloride values in sweat between patients with cystic fibrosis and normal control participants. A chloride concentration of greater than 60 mEq/L is diagnostic, values less than 40 are normal, and values between 40 and 60 are intermediate. Conditions other than cystic fibrosis can manifest an elevated sweat chloride including adrenal insufficiency, ectodermal dysplasia, nephrogenic diabetes insipidus, hypothyroidism, and malnutrition.

204. The answer is b. (*Behrman, 16/e, pp. 1309–1310. McMillan, 3/e, pp. 1227–1230. Rudolph, 20/e, pp. 1650–1652.*) The x-ray reveals a lung abscess involving the right upper lobe characterized by the round density, the air–fluid level, and the opaque rim. Lung abscesses are usually caused by anaerobic bacteria such as bacteroides, fusobacteria, and anaerobic streptococci, and on occasion by *Staphylococcus aureus* and *Klebsiella*. The organisms were previously sensitive to penicillin but some anaerobic organisms (especially bacteroides) are now resistant due to ß lactam production. Lung abscesses frequently respond surprisingly well to treatment with antibiotics alone.

205. The answer is d. (*Behrman, 16/e, pp. 2169–2170, McMillan, 3/e, pp. 621–625. Rudolph, 20/e, pp. 833–834, 847–849.*) Hydrocarbons with low viscosity and high volatility are the most likely agents to cause respiratory symptoms. Gasoline, kerosene, and furniture polish (which contain hydrocarbons) are common agents responsible for hydrocarbon aspiration. Motor oil, castor oil, and mineral oil can cause respiratory problems, but are less likely to do so because they are more viscous and have lower volatility. Hydrocarbon aspiration can produce dyspnea, cyanosis, and respiratory failure. Treatment is symptomatic. Oil of wintergreen is a highly concentrated form of salicylate that can cause symptoms of salicylate poisoning rather than pneumonitis.

206. The answer is d. *(Behrman, 16/e, pp. 885–897. McMillan, 3/e, pp. 1026–1039. Rudolph, 20/e, pp. 614–623.)* The key to controlling tuberculosis in children and eradicating the disease is early detection and appropriate treatment of adult cases, since the child, once infected, is at lifelong risk for the development of the disease and for infecting others unless given isoniazid prophylaxis. The usual source of the disease is an infected adult. Household contacts of a person with newly diagnosed active disease have a considerable risk of developing active tuberculosis and the risk is greatest for infants and children. Therefore, when tuberculosis is diagnosed in a child, the immediate family and close contacts should be tested with tuberculin skin tests and chest radiographs and treated appropriately when indicated. Bronchoscopy would be indicated only in unusual circumstances. Three to eight weeks is required after exposure before hypersensitivity to tuberculin develops. This means that the tuberculin test must be repeated in exposed persons if there is a negative reaction at the time that contact with the source of infection is broken. TB skin tests are usually negative in infants of this age, even when active disease is ongoing. A logical preventive measure is the administration of isoniazid to the baby for 3 months when a Mantoux (PPD) can then be placed. Transmission of tuberculosis occurs when bacilli-laden, small-sized droplets are dispersed into the air by the cough or sneeze of an infected adult. Small children with primary pulmonary tuberculosis are not considered infectious to others and they are not capable of coughing up and producing sputum. Sputum, when produced, is promptly swallowed, and for this reason, specimens for microbial confirmation can be obtained by means of gastric lavage from smaller children.

207. The answer is e. *(Behrman, 16/e, pp. 885–897. McMillan, 3/e, pp. 1026–1039. Rudolph, 20/e, pp. 614–623.)* The tuberculin skin test is based on the detection of delayed hypersensitivity to the antigen of *Mycobacterium tuberculosis*. Two to ten weeks after infection, the intradermal injection of antigen will result in a positive response indicated by induration. The tine test, a multipuncture skin test used widely for mass screening because of its ease of administration, uses a plastic unit with four stainless steel blades treated with a crude filtrate of culture medium containing old tuberculin (OT). The tine test has a number of problems, such as no standardization and variable results. Their use is discouraged, especially if TB is suspected. Retesting positive or doubtful tine reactions with the Mantoux test is indicated. The Mantoux intracutaneous tuberculin test uses a protein precipitate derived from OT (purified protein derivative, PPD) and is the preferred skin test. It is a more reliable test because of the efforts used in its preparation to standardize and preserve potency and because it delivers a defined amount of the antigen. The most appropriate next step in managing an asymptomatic, thriving child with a positive tine test is to administer a Mantoux test.

208. The answer is a. (*Behrman, 16/e, pp. 1259–1260. McMillan, 3/e, p. 639. Rudolph, 20/e, p. 460.*) Small children frequently introduce any number of small objects into their nose ranging from food to small toys. Initially, only local irritation occurs. Later, as prolonged obstruction is seen, symptoms increase to include worsening of pain, and a purulent, malodorous, bloody discharge can be seen. Unilateral nasal discharge in the presence of obstruction suggests the need to examine the patient for a nasal foreign body.

209. The answer is d. (*Behrman, 16/e, pp. 1268–1271. McMillan, 3/e, pp. 1256–1258. Rudolph, 20/e, pp. 1594–1595.*) Administration of steroids, a nasopharyngeal airway, the use of nasal CPAP, and tonsillectomy and adenoidectomy can be effective treatments for obstructive sleep apnea. Irradiation should not be used for fear of development of malignancy, particularly of the thyroid.

210. The answer is b. (*Behrman, 16/e, pp. 764, 795, 1330–1331. McMillan, 3/e, pp. 1010, 1229–1230. Rudolph, 20/e, pp. 1651–1652.*) Tension pneumothorax, a well-recognized complication of staphylococcal pneumonia, can be quickly lethal and is easily treated. This makes a high index of suspicion and prompt diagnosis mandatory. The other complications can occur also but do not require as prompt a response. Immediate action to relieve the tension is mandatory. This can be done by inserting a needle or catheter into the second or third intercostal spaces in the midclavicular line, with the patient supine. A three-way stopcock on the syringe is an added refinement.

211. The answer is e. *(Behrman, 16/e, pp. 1267–1268. McMillan, 3/e, pp. 1298–1299. Rudolph, 20/e, pp. 966–967.)* The only absolute indication for tonsillectomy is the need to rule out tumor (and perhaps severe aerodigestive obstruction). Many other indications have been proposed and many illnesses attributed to enlarged tonsils. Most tonsils that are considered too large are actually of normal size and reflect normal physiologic development. The usefulness of tonsillectomy to control such illnesses as recurrent streptococcal pharyngitis, otitis media, and upper respiratory infection is questionable and in some cases the procedure has proved to be unhelpful. In general, the decision to remove tonsils should be made on symptoms such as hypertrophy, obstruction, and chronic infection of the tonsillar tissue and not on symptoms at more distant sites.

212. The answer is d. *(Behrman, 16/e, pp. 1275–1276. McMillan, 3/e, pp. 572, 997, 1093, 1310. Rudolph, 20/e, pp. 576, 675, 1633.)* In the past, this disease was most commonly caused by invasive *Haemophilus influenzae* type B. Due to the widespread use of the Hib vaccine, this condition is now more commonly caused by group A beta hemolytic streptococcus, *M. catarrhalis,* or *S. pneumoniae*. Epiglottitis is a life-threatening form of infection-produced upper airway obstruction. The course of the illness is brief and prodromal symptoms are lacking. There is a sudden onset of sore throat, high fever, and prostration that is out of proportion to the duration of the illness. Drooling and difficulty in swallowing, a muffled voice, and preference for a characteristic sitting posture with the neck hyperextended may be noted. Unless preparations are available for immediate intubation by skilled personnel, any attempt to visualize the epiglottis should be avoided. Morbidity and mortality are usually related to a delay in establishing an airway early in the disease. Therefore, radiography of the neck, which may delay definitive treatment, is unwise.

213. The answer is c. *(Behrman, 16/e, p. 1068, McMillan, 3/e, pp. 1199–1202. Rudolph, 20/e, pp. 715–716.)* The presentation described is characteristic of visceral larva migrans from infestation with a common parasite of dogs, *Toxocara canis*. Dirt-eating children ingest the infectious ova. The larvae penetrate the intestine and migrate to visceral sites, such as the liver, lung, and brain, but do not return to the intestine, so the stools do not contain the ova or parasites. The diagnosis can be made by a specific enzyme-linked immunosorbent assay (ELISA) for *Toxocara*.

214. The answer is b. *(Behrman, 16/e, pp. 955–956. McMillan, 3/e, pp. 1278–1284. Rudolph, 20/e, p. 1264.)* Maxillary and ethmoid sinuses are large enough to harbor infections from infancy. Frontal sinuses are rarely large enough to harbor infections until the 6th to 10th year of life. Sphenoid sinuses do not become large until about the 3rd to 5th year of life. In general, a cold lasting longer than 10 to 14 days with fever and facial pain is indicative of sinusitis. Examination of the nose can reveal pus draining from the middle meatus in maxillary, frontal, or anterior ethmoid sinusitis. Pus in the superior meatus indicates sphenoid or posterior ethmoid sinuses. Diagnosis is on clinical grounds and can be difficult. Positive findings on plain sinus films in a symptomatic child are supportive of sinusitis. CT scans are more sensitive, but are usually reserved for the more complicated cases. The treatment is usually oral antibiotics for 10 to 14 days. Decongestants and antihistamines have not been shown to be helpful or necessary.

215. The answer is d. *(Behrman, 16/e, pp. 1275–1278. McMillan, 3/e, pp. 1307–1311. Rudolph, 20/e, pp. 672–677.)* The signs of illness described are those involving the airway above the point at which the trachea enters the neck and leaves the thorax, as in croup syndrome. Intrathoracic airway diseases, such as asthma or bronchiolitis, produce breathing difficulty on expiration with expiratory wheezing, prolonged expiration, and signs of air trapping due to the increased narrowing during expiration as the airways are exposed to the same intrathoracic pressure changes as the alveoli. The extrathoracic airway, to the contrary, tends to collapse on inspiration, producing the characteristic findings this patient demonstrates.

Agents causing croup include parainfluenza types I and III, influenza A and B, RSV, and occasionally, other viruses. Treatment is usually supportive but racemic epinephrine and corticosteroids reduce the length of time in the emergency room and hospitalizations.

216. The answer is e. *(Behrman, 16/e, p. 656. McMillan, 3/e, pp. 575, 2044. Rudolph, 20/e, p. 793.)* Therapeutic serum levels of theophylline are 10 to 20 µg/mL. Below these levels, a therapeutic effect may not be obtained and above them, toxicity supervenes with nausea, vomiting, cardiac arrhythmias, convulsions, and death. The narrow therapeutic window, its possible relationship to increased morbidity when combined with some beta agonists, and low efficacy, have reduced this drug's popularity. Nonetheless, it is important to know the effects of prescribing additional drugs for patients taking theophylline and of giving theophylline to patients taking these drugs. Erythromycin and cimetidine decrease the clearance of theophylline and increase its serum levels. Phenytoin and rifampin have the opposite effect. Penicillin has no effect on theophylline levels.

217. The answer is e. (*Behrman, 16/e, pp. 762–765, 795, 885–897, 914–915. McMillan, 3/e, pp. 893–894, 1026–1039, 1227–1230. Rudolph, 20/e, pp. 576, 614–623, 686–688, 1650–1652.*) Infections with *Mycoplasma pneumoniae* are common in older children and young adults. Although the infection typically produces lower-lobe bronchopneumonia, its effects are characteristically nonspecific and it can produce lobar pneumonia as well. It can produce upper respiratory infection, pharyngitis, otitis media and externa, bronchiolitis, hemolytic anemia, and Guillain-Barré syndrome. Treatment of choice is a macrolide antibiotic. *Staphylococcus aureus* is seen in infants less than 6 months of age; *Haemophilus influenza* is rarely seen with the wide spread use of *H. influenzae* B vaccine. At this age, *Mycobacterium tuberculosis* presents with hilar adenopathy and localized bronchu lobar pneumonia in the upper lobe most typically, and *S. pneumoniae* causes the sudden onset of high fever and a lobar pneumonia, often with pleural effusion. A TB skin test for this patient would be a good idea.

218. The answer is b. (*Behrman, 16/e, pp. 686–688. McMillan, 3/e, p. 2070. Rudolph, 20/e, p. 475.*) Treatment is similar to that of an insect sting in an allergic child. If respiratory distress is severe, intubation is necessary. Additional treatment can include bagging with oxygen and administration of epinephrine, plasma expanders, diphenhydramine, and cimetidine as indicated by the clinical course of the patient. Additional treatment such as administration of corticosteroids should be started early, but the effect will be delayed. Tourniquet therapy is not indicated and is potentially harmful.

219. The answer is e. (*Behrman, 16/e, pp. 1127–1128. Rudolph, 20/e, p. 1064.*) Many types of objects produce esophageal obstruction in young children, including small toys, coins, and food. Most are usually lodged below the cricopharyngeal muscle at the level of the aortic arch. Initially, the foreign body may cause a cough, drooling, and choking. Later, pain, avoidance of food (liquids are tolerated better), and shortness of breath can develop. Diagnosis is by history (as outlined in the question) and by radiographs (especially if the object is radiopaque). The usual treatment is removal of the object via esophagoscopy.

220–223. The answers are 220-e, 221-c, 222-a, 223-d. *(Behrman, 16/e, pp. 204–210, 743–744, 800–801, 1248–1250, 1479–1483. McMillan, 3/e, pp. 1450–1451. Rudolph, 20/e, pp. 1203–1207, 1327–1330, 1420.)* Fever, cough, and tachypnea in a patient with sickle cell anemia can be manifestations of pneumonia, pulmonary thromboemboli, or sepsis. Aside from being relatively common in patients with sickle cell anemia, these diseases can be rapidly progressive and quickly fatal. It is, therefore, important for the patient to be evaluated and treated on an emergency basis. The treatment requires hospitalization because it will almost certainly include systemic antibiotics, intravenous fluids, oxygen, and perhaps, blood transfusion.

In order to see cyanosis, there must be about 5 g of unoxygenated hemoglobin in the skin capillaries. In anemia this may not be possible as the total hemoglobin level can be beneath that. In addition, dark skin pigmentation and poor lighting contribute to making cyanosis an unreliable negative sign. With anemia and pulmonary disease, it should be assumed that the patient has impaired oxygenation.

The low pH in the arterial blood can be called acidemia. In this context, it is likely that the hydrogen ions come from lactic acid produced by anaerobic metabolism in tissues with inadequate oxygen delivery. Inadequate oxygenation is caused by the low PO_2, the low oxygen-carrying capacity of the blood (Hb 5 g/dL), and circulatory inadequacy due to the sickling itself and to the vascular disease it produces. The low PCO_2 reflects the hyperventilation, which is secondary to the respiratory difficulty, and to the anemia, and is also respiratory compensation for the metabolic acidosis.

Administration of 100% oxygen will rapidly raise alveolar oxygen concentration and in the absence of substantial right-to-left shunting of blood, will fully saturate the arterial hemoglobin. It will also dissolve 0.003 mL of oxygen per mm Hg of oxygen partial pressure in each deciliter of blood. This will serve to decrease the tissue hypoxia and increase the concentration of mixed venous oxygen, which may decrease the amount of sickling. The other choices are all undesirable or contraindicated.

224. The answer is c. *(Behrman, 16/e, p. 1266. McMillan, 3/e, pp. 572–573, 1299–1301. Rudolph, 20/e, p. 1634.)* Suppurative infection of the chain of lymph nodes between the posterior pharyngeal wall and the preverte-bral fascia leads to retropharyngeal abscesses. The most common causative organisms are *S. aureus*, group A ß-hemolytic streptococci, and oral anaer-obes. Presenting signs and symptoms include a history of pharyngitis, abrupt onset of fever with severe sore throat, refusal of food, drooling, and muffled or noisy breathing. A bulge in the posterior pharyngeal wall is diagnostic, as are radiographs of the lateral neck that reveal the retropha-ryngeal mass. Palpation (with adequate provision for emergency control of the airway in case of rupture) reveals a fluctuant mass. Treatment should include incision and drainage if fluctuans is present.

225-226. The answers are 225-d, 226-e. (*Behrman, 16/e, p. 920. McMillan, 3/e, pp. 451–453, 896–897. Rudolph, 20/e, pp. 562–563, 1654–1655.*) Chlamydiae, sexually transmitted among adults, are spread to infants dur-ing birth from genitally infected mothers. The sites of infection in infants are the lungs and the conjunctivae, where chlamydiae cause afebrile pneu-monia and inclusion conjunctivitis, respectively, in infants between 2 and 12 weeks of age. Diagnosis is confirmed by culture of secretions and by antibody titers. In adolescents, chlamydial infections may be a cause of cervicitis, salpingitis, endometritis, and epididymitis and appear to be an important cause of tubal infertility. The most common treatment for this condition includes macrolide antibiotics orally, which clears both the naso-pharyngeal secretions when a conjunctivitis is present and prevents the pneumonia that can occur later.

227. The answer is b. (*Behrman, 16/e, pp. 1279–1282. McMillan, 3/e, pp. 570–571, 640. Rudolph, 20/e, pp. 1635–1638.*) Recurrent pneumonias in an otherwise healthy child should indicate the potential for anatomic blockage of an airway. In the patient in this question, the findings on clin-ical examination suggest a foreign body in the airway. Inspiratory and expiratory films can be helpful. Routine inspiratory films are likely to appear normal or near normal (as outlined in the question). Expiratory films will identify air trapping behind the foreign body. It is uncommon for the foreign body to be visible on the plain radiograph; a high index of suspicion is necessary to make the diagnosis. Suspected foreign bodies in the airway are potentially diagnosed with fluoroscopy, but rigid broncho-scopy is not only diagnostic but also the treatment of choice for removal of the foreign body.

228–230. The answers are 228-c, 229-d, 230-b. (*Behrman, 16/e, pp. 204–210, 1248–1250. Rudolph, 20/e, pp. 1329–1330, 1324–1325, 1611–1613, 1630.*) The laboratory results of row (C) indicate a striking respiratory alkalosis. This could be secondary to voluntary hyperventilation or inappropriate respirator settings for a patient on a ventilator and is also typical of acute hyperventilation syndrome secondary to anxiety. Such a patient can complain of dyspnea, chest pain, tingling, and dizziness and can even have generalized convulsions secondary to low ionized calcium levels. Rebreathing into a paper bag can be both therapeutic and diagnostic.

The blood gases of row (D) are the only ones given that are relatively normal except for a low oxygen partial pressure. The mild respiratory alkalosis and metabolic acidosis can be a consequence of the hypoxia. These results could be obtained in a patient with moderately severe pneumonia, bronchiolitis, or asthma, secondary to ventilation-perfusion inequality, with some areas of the lung underventilated with respect to perfusion. This cause of hypoxia can be easily corrected by giving the patient relatively small increases in oxygen concentration to breathe. These results would also be typical of findings in patients with right-to-left shunting of blood, as in tetralogy of Fallot. In which case, giving oxygen would not help (but cardiac surgery was not one of the options given to you in this question).

The results in row (A) show fairly severe metabolic acidosis with respiratory compensation and without hypoxia. These would be typical for someone in early shock and would most commonly be seen in children with diarrhea. Treatment of this type of acidosis is hydration.

The blood gases of row (B) demonstrate an uncompensated respiratory acidosis with hypoxia but with no metabolic acidosis. This is compatible with acute hypoventilation, which could be produced by a tension pneumothorax, for example. This can be treated easily by placing a needle or catheter in the pleural space and evacuating the air.

231–234. The answers are 231-a, 232-c, 233-b, 234-d. (*Behrman, 16/e, pp. 204–210, 1248–1250, 1267–1268. Rudolph, 20/e, pp. 967, 1329–1330, 1594– 1596, 1630.*) The data on row (A) indicate severe acidemia and severe hypoxia with a marked respiratory acidosis and metabolic acidosis. These are manifestations of severe ventilatory failure, probably accompanied by circulatory failure or cardiac arrest. This mandates the most aggressive therapy, including assisted ventilation with administration of high oxygen levels. Other measures to restore circulation and improve the acidemia are also indicated.

The results of row (C) show metabolic alkalosis. The high P_{CO_2} and low P_{O_2} result from compensatory hypoventilation. This can all be secondary to excessive body potassium losses from diuretics.

The results in row (B) indicate respiratory acidosis with metabolic compensation, indicating chronic upper airway obstruction. A common cause of chronic hypoventilation in children is hypertrophied tonsils and adenoids, which may be an indication for tonsillectomy or adenoidectomy (or both).

The blood gases of row (D) are impossible in a patient breathing room air. The P_{CO_2} cannot go up without the P_{O_2} dropping roughly proportionately. An increase in P_{CO_2} of 20 mm Hg from 40 to 60 mm Hg should, therefore, produce a fall in P_{O_2} from 90 to 70 mm Hg. The test should be repeated after the blood gas equipment has been checked and recalibrated.

THE GASTROINTESTINAL TRACT

Questions

DIRECTIONS: Each item below contains a question or incomplete statement followed by suggested responses. Select the **one best** response to each question.

235. A 4-year-old boy presents with a history of constipation since the age of 6 months. His stools, produced every 3 to 4 days, are described as large and hard. Physical examination is normal; rectal examination reveals a large ampulla, poor sphincter tone, and stool in the rectal vault. The next step in the management of this infant would be

a. lower GI barium study
b. parental reassurance and counseling
c. serum electrolyte measurement
d. upper GI barium study
e. initiation of synthroid

236. A 10-year-old boy has been having belly aches for about 2 years. They occur at night as well as during the day. Occasionally, he vomits after the onset of pain. Occult blood has been found in his stool. His father also gets frequent stomach aches. The most likely diagnosis is

a. peptic ulcer
b. appendicitis
c. Meckel's diverticulum
d. intussusception
e. pinworm infestation

237. A 5-year-old child is noted to be iron deficient. Upon questioning his family, they report several episodes of grossly bloody (maroon) stools. Which of the following is a likely explanation for his anemia?

a. increased demands for iron due to accelerated growth
b. Meckel's diverticulum
c. infestation by hookworm
d. peptic ulcer
e. recurrent epistaxis

238. A 6-month-old infant has large, foul-smelling stools and is not gaining weight. Sweat chloride level was 68. Appropriate nutritional recommendations include

a. supplementation with water-soluble vitamins
b. pancreatic enzyme replacement
c. high fat diet
d. low protein diet
e. low carbohydrate diet

239. A 1-week-old previously healthy infant presents to the emergency room with the acute onset of bilious vomiting. The abdominal plain film shows dilated proximal loops of bowel and stomach. Barium enema reveals the cecum to be in the left lower quadrant. The most likely diagnosis for this patient is

a. jejunal atresia
b. hypertrophic pyloric stenosis
c. malrotation of the intestines with volvulus
d. appendicitis
e. intussusception

240. A 14-month-old infant receives chronic total parenteral nutrition for short gut syndrome. Which of the following is the most common complication?

a. sepsis
b. liver disease
c. pulmonary emboli
d. air emboli
e. irreversible atrophy of the mucosa of the small intestine

241. A 4-week-old boy presents with a 10-day history of vomiting that has increased in frequency and forcefulness. The vomitus is not bile stained. The child feeds avidly and looks well, but he has been losing weight. An ultrasound of the abdomen is shown. The most likely diagnosis is

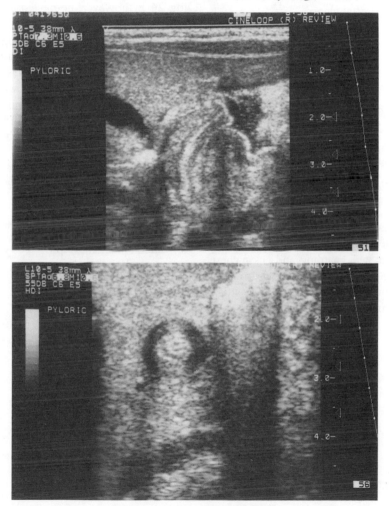

(Courtesy Susan John, M.D.)

a. pyloric stenosis
b. small intestinal obstruction
c. gastroenteritis
d. intussusception
e. brain tumor

242. The correct statement regarding Hirschsprung's disease is

a. fecal soiling is common
b. definitive diagnosis requires rectal biopsy
c. rectal manometry usually is normal
d. once diagnosis is established, a trial of medical therapy such as high fiber diet is indicated
e. enterocolitis is a common finding but rarely serious

243. A 14-year-old boy has sickle cell disease. He presents to the emergency room with the complaints of increased jaundice, abdominal pain, nausea, vomiting, and fever. His examination is remarkable for jaundice, pain of the right upper quadrant with guarding, and a clear chest. Chest radiographs appear normal. The test most likely to reveal the cause of this pain is

a. serum chemistries
b. complete blood count with platelets and differential
c. ultrasound of the right upper quadrant
d. upper GI series
e. hepatitis panel

244. An 8-year-old is accidentally hit in the abdomen by a baseball bat. After several minutes of discomfort, he seems to be fine. Over the ensuing 24 h, however, he develops a fever, abdominal pain radiating to the back, and persistent vomiting. On examination, the child appears quite uncomfortable. The abdomen is tender with decreased bowel sounds throughout, but especially painful with guarding in the midepigastric region. The test likely to confirm your suspicions is

a. serum amylase
b. complete blood count with differential and platelets
c. serum total and direct bilirubin levels
d. abdominal radiograph
e. electrolyte panel

245. A 10-month-old boy, recently arrived from Guyana, has a 5-h history of crying with intermittent drawing up of his knees to his chest. On the way to the emergency room he passes a loose, bloody stool. He has had no vomiting and has refused his bottle since the crying began. Physical examination is noteworthy for an irritable infant whose abdomen is very difficult to examine because of constant crying. His temperature is 38.8°C (101.8°F). The rectal ampulla is empty but there is some gross blood on the examining finger. The most helpful study in the immediate management of this patient would be

a. stool culture
b. examination of the stool for ova and parasites
c. an air contrast enema
d. examination of the blood smear
e. coagulation studies

246. A 12-month-old girl has been spitting up her meals since 1 month of age. Her growth is at the 95th percentile and she is otherwise asymptomatic and without findings on physical examination. The most likely diagnosis is

a. pyloric stenosis
b. partial duodenal atresia
c. hypothyroidism
d. gastroesophageal reflux disease
e. tracheoesophageal fistula

247. A 14-year-old girl has a 9-month history of diarrhea, abdominal pain (usually periumbilical and postprandial), fever, and weight loss. She has had several episodes of blood in her stools. Which of the following is the most likely diagnosis in this child?

a. chronic appendicitis
b. chronic pancreatitis
c. Crohn's disease
d. bulimia
e. gallstones

248. A 6-month-old infant has eaten a diet with the following content and intake for the past 5 months: protein 4 percent of calories, fat 50 percent of calories, carbohydrates 46 percent of calories, calories 105 per kilogram of body weight per day. The patient's disturbance is

a. rickets
b. marasmus
c. obesity
d. tetany
e. kwashiorkor

249. An 8-month-old child regularly regurgitates a large portion of her feeds. In the diagnostic evaluation of gastroesophageal reflux for this infant, the LEAST helpful procedure is

a. barium swallow and upper GI series
b. urea breath test
c. esophageal manometry
d. esophageal pH probe
e. technetium 99m scintiscan

250. Although the most common complication of a Meckel's diverticulum is painless rectal bleeding, which of the following is also a common presentation of this condition?

a. meconium ileus
b. rectal prolapse
c. obstruction of the common bile duct
d. hepatosplenomegaly
e. intussusception

251. Which of the following studies is helpful in the diagnosis of lactose intolerance?

a. barium swallow and upper GI
b. hydrogen excretion in breath after oral administration of lactose
c. esophageal manometry
d. technetium 99m scintiscan
e. pH probe of the esophagus

252. A 6-week-old infant is admitted to the hospital with jaundice. Her outpatient blood work demonstrated a total bilirubin of 12 mg/dL with a direct portion of 3.5 mg/dL. Which of the following disorders is likely to be responsible?

a. ABO incompatibility
b. choledochal cyst
c. Rh incompatibility
d. Gilbert's disease
e. Crigler-Najjar syndrome

253. An 11-year-old child has been diagnosed with hepatitis C infection. Which of the following may be considered in the treatment of chronic hepatitis C infection?

a. active vaccination
b. interferon
c. gamma globulin
d. zidovudine
e. low protein diet

254. An awake, alert infant with a 2-day history of diarrhea presents with a depressed fontanelle, tachycardia, sunken eyes, and the loss of skin elasticity. The appropriate percent of dehydration is

a. less than 1 percent
b. 1 percent to 5 percent
c. 5 percent to 9 percent
d. 10 percent to 15 percent
e. more than 20 percent

255. The correct statement regarding hypernatremic dehydration with Na+ in serum 170 mEq/L and 10 percent loss of body weight includes

a. no early evidence of low blood pressure
h need for rapid intravenous rehydration with 0.2% saline
c. inclusion of calcium gluconate in the IV fluid is advised
d. lethargy is common
e. delayed reintroduction of regular diet

256. An acceptable solution for oral rehydration of infants with moderately severe diarrhea presumably caused by *Escherichia coli* has the composition

a. Na+ 10 mEq/L, K+ 15 mEq/L, Cl− 25 mEq/L
b. Na+ 90 mEq/L, K+ 15 mEq/L, Cl− 75 mEq/L, HCO₃− 30 mEq/L, glucose 111 mmol/L (2 g/dL)
c. Na+ 90 mEq/L, K+ 15 mEq/L, Cl− 75 mEq/L, HCO₃− 30 mEq/L, glucose 333 mmol/L (6 g/dL)
d. Na+200 mEq/L, K+ 15 mEq/L, Cl− 135 mEq/L, HCO₃− 30 mEq/L, glucose 111 mmol/L (2 g/dL)
e. glucose 5 g/dL in isotonic saline (Na+ 150 mEq/L, Cl− 150 mEq/L)

257. A mother of a 6-month-old infant is concerned that her baby may be teething. You explain to her that the first teeth to erupt in most children are the

a. mandibular central incisors
b. maxillary lateral incisors
c. maxillary first molars
d. mandibular cuspids (canines)
e. first premolars (bicuspids)

258. A 4-year-old child is noted to have extensive maxillary tooth decay (especially frontal) and posterior maxillary and mandibular decay. The mandibular frontal teeth are essentially normal. This characteristic pattern of tooth decay is due to

a. excessive use of fluoride
b. tetracycline
c. use of bottled water that lacks fluoride
d. caries from nursing with a baby bottle
e. consumption of too much candy

259. An 8-year-old boy is brought to your office with the complaint of abdominal pain. The pain is worse during the week and seems to be less prominent during the weekends and during the summer. The patient's growth and development are normal. The physical examination is unremarkable. Laboratory screening, including stool for guaiac, complete blood count, urinalysis, and chemistry panel, yields normal results. The next step in the care of this patient should be to

a.   perform an upper GI series
b.   perform CT of the abdomen
c.   administer a trial of H2 blockers
d.   observe the patient and reassure the patient and family
e.   recommend a lactose-free diet

260. A 55-day-old former 27-week premature infant is noted by the neonatal nurse to have a swelling in the left groin extending into the scrotum but not involving the testicle. The swelling is not tender, firm, hot, or red, and it does not transilluminate. It seems to resolve with pressure, but returns when the infant begins to perform the Valsalva maneuver. The most appropriate course of action at this point is to

a.   obtain a surgical consultation
b.   perform a needle aspiration
c.   order a barium enema
d.   order a KUB
e.   do nothing; spontaneous resolution will occur

261. A 12-year-old girl was hit in the face by a baseball 15 min earlier and has had her mandibular incisors knocked out. Which of the following represents an accurate plan of action?

a.   the teeth should be rinsed in hot water
b.   foreign matter adhering to the teeth should be immediately scrubbed off
c.   the teeth may be transported in tea, juice, or cola
d.   avulsed teeth can be transported in the mouth of the older, cooperative pediatric patient if they cannot be reinserted at the scene
e.   a dental appointment should be made within 72 hours

262. An 18-month-old infant is found with the contents of a bottle of drain cleaner in his mouth. A true statement concerning treatment for this caustic ingestion is

a.   emesis is the immediate emergency treatment
b.   endoscopic examination is indicated within the first 12 to 24 h
c.   decontamination by activated charcoal is effective
d.   neutralization by drinking a solution of the opposite pH is effective
e.   having the patient drink copious amounts of milk or water to dilute the caustic is essential

263. The use of activated charcoal would be LEAST effective in the emergency treatment of ingestion of which of the following?

a. phenobarbital
b. theophylline
c. ferrous sulfate
d. digitoxin
e. tricyclic antidepressants

DIRECTIONS: Each group of questions below consists of lettered options followed by numbered items. For each numbered item, select the appropriate lettered option(s). Each lettered option may be used once, more than once, or not at all. **Choose exactly the number of options indicated following each item.**

Items 264–268

For each description below, select the disorder with which it is most likely to be associated.

a. Peutz-Jeghers syndrome
b. Gardner's syndrome
c. juvenile colonic polyps
d. familial adenomatous polyposis
e. intestinal hemangioma

264. Intestinal lesions commonly show malignant degeneration
(SELECT 2 DISORDERS)

265. This disorder is associated with soft-tissue masses of the mandible
(SELECT 1 DISORDER)

266. Massive, even fatal, bleeding can occur
(SELECT 1 DISORDER)

267. Disorders that are usually not inherited
(SELECT 2 DISORDERS)

268. This is the most common tumor of bowel in childhood
(SELECT 1 DISORDER)

Items 269–274

For each characteristic, select the fluid that it most closely describes.

a. apple juice
b. whole cow's milk
c. oral rehydration solution (World Health Organization)
d. cola
e. human milk

269. The highest in carbohydrate concentration
(SELECT 1 FLUID)

270. The lowest in carbohydrate concentration
(SELECT 1 FLUID)

271. The highest in potassium concentration
(SELECT 1 FLUID)

272. The highest in sodium concentration
(SELECT 1 FLUID)

273. The highest in protein concentration
(SELECT 1 FLUID)

274. The lowest in calories
(SELECT 1 FLUID)

Items 275–278

For each description below, select the disorder with which it is most likely to be associated.

a. Behçet's disease
b. colic
c. short bowel syndrome
d. gluten-sensitive enteropathy
e. cystic fibrosis
f. Wolman's disease
g. Reye's syndrome

275. A 6-year-old child with vomiting, seizures, coma, and liver failure 6 days after a varicella infection
(SELECT 1 DISORDER)

276. Foul-smelling, bulky stools in a 3-month-old child with a history of failure to thrive
(SELECT 1 DISORDER)

277. A 1-month-old otherwise healthy child with daily periods of increased crying, fussiness, and passage of flatus during the evening hours
(SELECT 1 DISORDER)

278. An irritable 8-month-old child with diarrhea and poor weight gain each time cereal is introduced into his diet
(SELECT 1 DISORDER)

THE GASTROINTESTINAL TRACT

Answers

235. The answer is b. *(Behrman, 16/e, pp. 1105, 1138–1141. McMillan, 3/e, pp. 313–315, 1637–1639, 2281–2282. Rudolph, 20/e, pp. 1038–1041, 1115–1117.)* Hirschsprung's disease is usually suspected in the chronically constipated child despite the fact that 98 percent of such children have functional constipation. Finding a dilated, stool-filled anal canal with poor tone on the physical examination of a well-grown child supports the diagnosis of functional constipation. The difficulty in treating functional constipation once it has been established emphasizes the need for prompt identification and treatment of problems with defecation and for counseling of parents regarding proper toileting behavior. The extensive workup of this patient would likely be negative and expensive and is not indicated.

236. The answer is a. *(Behrman, 16/e, pp. 1147–1150. McMillan, 3/e, pp. 1195, 1642–1655, 1702–1704. Rudolph, 20/e, pp. 717–719, 1070–1072, 1090–1091, 1105–1106.)* The presence of nocturnal abdominal pain and gastrointestinal bleeding and a positive family history support a diagnosis of peptic ulcer disease. Pain is the most common symptom. Symptoms often persist for several years before diagnosis. The increased incidence of peptic ulcer disease in families (25 percent to 50 percent) and concordance in monozygotic twins suggest a genetic basis for the disease. Antibiotic treatment for *Helicobacter pylori* in patients not responding to conventional therapy can cure this disease in some patients. Appendicitis and intussusception are acute events. Pinworms produce perianal pruritus but do not commonly cause abdominal pain or other serious problems. Meckel's diverticulum causes painless rectal bleeding, usually during early childhood.

237. The answer is b. *(Behrman, 16/e, pp. 1065–1066, 1137–1138, 1147–1150, 1260, 1469–1471. McMillan, 3/e, pp. 1447–1448, 1642–1652. Rudolph, 20/e, pp. 719–720, 958, 1070, 1090–1091, 1176–1180.)* Iron deficiency is most common between 6 months and 3 years of age. During this period, the need for iron is increased because of accelerated growth, and this need is often not met when the diet consists predominantly of cow's milk, a uniquely iron-poor food. Growth plateaus during the preschool and pre-adolescent years and the mixed diets of children in this period are more likely to provide them with adequate iron. Chronic loss of blood from the intestinal tract or from nosebleeds can quickly deplete the iron stores of children. In adolescence, there are increased requirements for iron because of rapid growth. The adolescent female has the additional risk of becoming iron-deficient from the loss of menstrual blood.

Grossly positive blood in the stool of this patient requires a further evaluation. The Meckel's diverticulum results from an embryologic remnant of the vitelline duct. Gastric tissue in the area ulcerates causing intermittent bleeding. Blood can be microscopic or massive and grossly positive. The bleeding is often painless and is intermittent. The diverticulum can serve as a lead point for intussusception with resultant symptoms of obstruction. The diagnosis is with a Meckel scan (Tc-99m pertechnetate nuclear scan), which demonstrates a lesion in the right lower quadrant.

Hookworms are caused by two species of roundworm, *Necator americanus* and *Ancylostoma duodenale*. Symptoms include abdominal pain, weakness, dizziness, eosinophilia, pica, guaiac positive stools, and anemia. Gross bleeding and melena are rare.

Peptic ulcer disease often presents with epigastric pain, discomfort, vomiting, anorexia, early satiety, and weight loss. Bleeding is usually noted as hematemesis or melena. Bright red blood from the rectum is unusual without severe disease.

Epistaxis causes anemia of chronic blood loss, but the blood in the stool is usually only guaiac positive or is melanotic. Bright red blood from the rectum from nosebleeds is distinctly abnormal.

238. The answer is b. *(Behrman, 16/e, pp. 1315–1327. McMillan, 3/e, pp. 1242–1254. Rudolph, 20/e, pp. 1640–1650.)* The goal in treatment of patients with cystic fibrosis is to supply enough calories to maintain normal growth. Extra calories are needed to replace those lost as a result of gastrointestinal losses, to offset the catabolic and anorectic effects of respiratory infection, and for catch-up growth. Almost 90 percent of patients have poor digestion of fat and protein as a result of the deficiency of pancreatic function, which may be partially corrected by oral pancreatic enzyme replacement; protein and fat losses are reduced and patients are usually able to tolerate a reasonably normal diet. The high caloric density of fat is useful in meeting the patient's caloric needs. Supplementation with fat-soluble vitamins (A, D, E, and K) is necessary. With severe disease, feedings by nasogastric tube, percutaneous enterostomy, or intravenous nutrition can be necessary.

239. The answer is c. *(Behrman, 16/e, pp. 1135–1136. McMillan, 3/e, 311–312. Rudolph, 20/e, pp. 1067–1068.)* Malrotation results when incomplete rotation of the intestines occurs during embryologic development. The most common type of malrotation is failure of the cecum to move to its correct location in the right lower quadrant. Most patients present in the first weeks of life with bilious vomiting indicative of bowel obstruction and/or intermittent abdominal pain. Acute presentation, similar to that in the question, is caused by a volvulus of the intestines. The diagnosis is confirmed by radiographs; barium contrast studies (upper GI and/or enema) demonstrates malposition of the cecum in the vast majority of cases. Treatment is surgical.

240. The answer is a. *(Behrman, 16/e, p. 1165. McMillan, 3/e, p. 335. Rudolph, 20/e, pp. 1020–1025.)* Parenteral nutrition, particularly when a central line is used, has a relatively high risk of complications, so it should not be used without good indication. The most common complication, and one of the most serious, is sepsis (1 percent to 5 percent of patients). In addition to the complications mentioned, thrombosis of central veins, perforations of veins with infusion and bleeding into the pleural space and other sites, pneumothorax, brachial plexus injury, and skin sloughing can also occur. Small intestinal mucosal atrophy is reversed with oral feedings. Awareness of these complications and the practice of careful techniques may minimize the risks of this sometimes life-saving nutritional procedure.

241. The answer is a. *(Behrman, 16/e, pp. 1130–1131. McMillan, 3/e, p. 311. Rudolph, 20/e, p. 1068.)* A history of nonbilious vomiting of 10 days' duration in a child who does not look ill points to infantile hypertrophic pyloric stenosis as the most likely diagnosis. The ultrasound demonstrates the thickened pylorus. The incidence of this condition in infants is between 1:250 and 1:750, with males affected more often than females. Although there is no specific pattern of inheritance, a familial incidence has been observed in about 15 percent of patients. The prevalence of pyloric stenosis is possibly also higher in first-born infants. White infants have a higher incidence of pyloric stenosis than African-American and Asian infants. Metabolic alkalosis with low serum potassium and chloride levels is frequently seen in pyloric stenosis as a result of loss of gastric contents from vomiting.

242. The answer is b. *(Behrman, 16/e, pp. 1138–1141. McMillan, 3/e, pp. 313–315. Rudolph, 20/e, pp. 1115–1118.)* The diagnosis of Hirschsprung's disease should be suspected in a child with intractable chronic constipation without fecal soiling (approximately 3 percent have fecal soiling). In contrast, overflow diarrhea caused by leakage of the unformed fecal stream around a rectal impaction is common in functional constipation. A neonatal history of delayed passage of meconium is often obtained and the infant can continue to be constipated and to have bouts of abdominal distention and vomiting. The infant is also at risk of developing enterocolitis, a serious life-threatening consequence of the partial obstruction. Radiologic study by barium enema and rectal manometry are accurate diagnostic tools. Identification of an aganglionic segment of bowel by punch or suction biopsy can establish the diagnosis. Histochemical tissue examination showing increased amounts of acetylcholinesterase and an absence of ganglia cells is confirmatory. Rectal manometric studies have shown that in aganglionic megacolon, the usual relaxation of the internal rectal sphincter in response to balloon inflation does not occur. Surgery is indicated as soon as the diagnosis is made.

243. The answer is c. *(Behrman, 16/e, pp. 1213, 1479–1483. McMillan, 3/e, pp. 1450–1451, 1736–1737. Rudolph, 20/e, pp. 1203–1207.)* Cholecystitis and cholelithiasis are unusual diseases in children and are usually associated with predisposing disorders such as hemolytic anemia. Pain of the right upper quadrant, nausea, vomiting, fever, and jaundice are symptoms of acute cholecystitis. The diagnosis is confirmed with an ultrasound of the gallbladder.

244. The answer is a. *(Behrman, 16/e, pp. 1191–1193. McMillan, 3/e, pp. 1711–1712. Rudolph, 20/e, pp. 1120–1121.)* The causes of pancreatitis in children are varied, with about one fourth of cases without predisposing etiology and about one third of cases as a feature of another systemic disease. Traumatic cases are usually due to blunt trauma to the abdomen. Acute pancreatitis is difficult to diagnose; a high index of suspicion is necessary. Common clinical features include severe pain with nausea and vomiting. Tenderness, guarding or rebound pain, abdominal distention, and a paralytic ileus are signs and symptoms often seen. No diagnostic test is completely accurate. An elevated total serum amylase with the correct clinical history and signs and symptoms is the best diagnostic tool. Plain films of the abdomen exclude other diagnoses; ultrasonography of the pancreas can reveal enlargement of the pancreas, gallstones, cysts, and pseudocysts. Supportive care is indicated until the condition resolves.

245. The answer is c. (*Behrman, 16/e, pp. 1142–1143. McMillan, 3/e, pp. 1652–1655. Rudolph, 20/e, pp. 1071–1072.*) The usual presentation of intussusception is that of an infant between 4 and 10 months of age who has a sudden onset of intermittent colicky abdominal pain. The child can appear normal when the pain abates, but as it recurs with increasing frequency, the child can begin to vomit and become progressively more obtunded. The passage of stool containing blood and mucus, and resembling currant jelly, is often observed. Early examination of the abdomen can be unremarkable, but as the problem persists, a sausage-shaped mass in the right upper quadrant is frequently palpated. A contrast enema examination under fluoroscopic control can be therapeutic as well as diagnostic when the hydrostatic effects of the column of air serve to reduce the intussusception. Early diagnosis prevents bowel ischemia. The cause of most intussusceptions is unknown, but a Meckel's diverticulum or polyp can serve as a lead point.

246. The answer is d. (*Behrman, 16/e, pp. 1125–1126. McMillan, 3/e, pp. 320–321. Rudolph, 20/e, pp. 1058–1062.*) Gastroesophageal reflux is a common pediatric complaint, common in the first 1 to 2 months of age and resolving in the first 1 to 2 years of life. About 7 percent of children have reflux severe enough to come to medical attention, and only 2 percent of that group requires investigation. For most children, conservative treatment (small feeds, thickened formula, avoiding high fat meals, etc.) suffice. A smaller number need pharmacologic therapy; and an even smaller number require surgery.

247. The answer is c. (*Behrman, 16/e, pp. 1150–1151. McMillan, 3/e, pp. 1674–1681. Rudolph, 20/e, pp. 1097–1099.*) The presentation of Crohn's depends on the location and extent of lesions. Onset of the gastrointestinal or extraintestinal symptoms is insidious. The common presentation is as described. Crohn's disease (granulomatous colitis) characteristically is associated with transmural, granulomatous intestinal lesions that are discontinuous and can appear in both the small and large intestine. Although Crohn's disease can first appear as a rectal fissure or fistula, the rectum is often spared. Arthritis/arthralgia occurs in a minority (11 percent) of affected children. Other extraintestinal symptoms include erythema nodosum or pyoderma gangrenosum, liver disease, renal calculi, uveitis, anemia, specific nutrient deficiency, and growth failure. In relation to the general population, the risk of colonic carcinoma in affected persons is increased but not nearly to the degree associated with ulcerative colitis.

248. The answer is e. *(Behrman, 16/e, pp. 169–171. McMillan, 3/e, p. 1472. Rudolph, 20/e, pp. 1005–1006, 1015–1016.)* The syndrome of kwashiorkor is caused by a diet that is deficient in protein leading to low serum albumin, which causes decreased plasma volume and increased interstitial fluid or edema. The term marasmus refers to a combined inadequacy of protein and energy in which the deficiency is dominated by the lack of food in general. The minimum requirement for protein is 8 percent of the total daily calories when the protein provided is from high-quality animal sources. These patients have a high death rate from intercurrent infections.

249. The answer is b. *(Behrman, 16/e, pp. 1125–1126. McMillan, 3/e, pp. 320–321, 958. Rudolph, 20/e, pp. 1058–1062.)* Barium swallow and upper GI series are helpful in detecting anatomic abnormalities such as antral web, pyloric stenosis, malrotation, and annular pancreas. To confirm the presence of gastroesophageal reflux (GER), the best test is the esophageal pH probe, which measures the frequency and duration of falls in pH, thereby indicating acid reflux. Esophageal manometry is used to identify poor tone of the lower esophageal sphincter. Delayed gastric emptying as well as evidence of aspiration can be demonstrated by use of a technetium 99m scintiscan. Chest x-ray can show the effects of aspiration, that is, evidence of a pulmonary infiltration. The urea breath test is an indirect method of establishing the presence of *Helicobacter pylori*, the organism considered to be causally related to peptic ulcer disease. The test measures labeled CO_2 exhaled after ingestion of labeled ^{13}C or ^{14}C urea, thereby identifying large amounts of urease produced by the organism. Urease converts urea to ammonia, which may act as a cytotoxin to gastric mucosa and lead to ulceration. The urea breath test is not used in the workup of GER.

250. The answer is e. *(Behrman, 16/e, pp. 1137–1138. McMillan, 3/e, pp. 1652–1654. Rudolph, 20/e, pp. 1071–1072.)* The embryonic duct connecting the yolk sac to the intestine can fail to regress completely and persist as a diverticulum attached to the ileum. The lining of this Meckel's diverticulum usually contains acid-secreting gastric mucosa that can produce ulcerations of the diverticulum itself or the adjacent ileum. Bleeding, perforation, or diverticulitis can occur. The diverticulum can lead to volvulus of itself and of the small intestine and it can also undergo eversion and intussusception. Diagnosis can be made by technetium scan and treatment is by surgical excision.

251. The answer is b. *(Behrman, 16/e, pp. 1168, 1175–1176. McMillan, 3/e, pp. 1698–1699. Rudolph, 20/e, pp. 1083–1085.)* Upper GI/barium swallow and measurement of esophageal pH is useful in the diagnosis of gastroesophageal reflux. Lactase is a disaccharidase localized in the brush border of the intestinal villous cells. It hydrolyzes lactose to its constituent monosaccharides, glucose and galactose. Intestinal lactase levels are usually normal at birth in all populations; however, lactase deficiency is a common, genetically predetermined condition. Sucrose, also a disaccharide, is a nonreducing sugar composed of glucose and fructose that is hydrolyzed by the brush border enzyme sucrase. Lactase activity is not readily increased by the oral administration of substrate or the inclusion of lactose in the diet. The clinical symptoms of lactose malabsorption are due to the presence of osmotically active, undigested lactose, which may act to increase intestinal fluid volume, alter transit time, and produce the symptoms of abdominal cramps, distention, and, occasionally, watery diarrhea. Bacterial metabolism of the nonabsorbed carbohydrates in the colon to carbon dioxide and hydrogen may contribute to the clinical symptoms. Acquired lactase deficiency is often associated with conditions of the gastrointestinal tract that cause intestinal mucosal injury (e.g., sprue and regional enteritis).

Diagnostic techniques for lactose intolerance include removal of the offending sugar with a reproduction of symptoms upon reintroduction. Although the ingestion of even small amounts of lactose can be diagnostic if gastrointestinal symptoms occur, the measurement of breath hydrogen is more specific as it is not affected by glucose metabolism or gastric emptying. Similarly, an acidic stool pH in the presence of reducing substances would be diagnostic. Direct measurement of enzyme levels combined with histologic evaluation helps to differentiate an acquired (secondary versus primary) lactase deficiency in which the intestinal histology is normal.

252. The answer is b. *(Behrman, 16/e, pp. 1198–1201. McMillan, 3/e, pp. 205–206, 315–319. Rudolph, 20/e, p. 1136.)* Obstructive jaundice (i.e., direct-reacting bilirubin greater than 20 percent of the total) requires investigation in all infants. Cystic fibrosis and alpha1-antitrypsin deficiency should be considered in the diagnostic evaluation of any child with obstructive jaundice. Other diseases to be excluded include galactosemia, tyrosinemia, and urinary tract or other infections, including toxoplasmosis, cytomegalovirus, rubella, syphilis, and herpesvirus. Ultrasound examination to rule out choledochal cyst may be included with a ^{99}Tc hepatic imiodiacetic acid (HIDA) scan to assess the patency of the biliary tree. Liver biopsy can assist in the diagnosis by providing a histologic diagnosis (e.g., hepatitis), tissue for enzyme activity (i.e., inborn error of metabolism), or tissue for microscopic determination of storage diseases. ABO and Rh incompatibility could cause direct hyperbilirubinemia if there were brisk hemolysis at birth, which would then lead to inspissated bile syndrome. All of the other causes listed typically lead to indirect hyperbilirubinemia.

253. The answer is b. *(Behrman, 16/e, pp. 773–776. McMillan, 3/e, pp. 449, 1726. Rudolph, 20/e, pp. 650–651.)* Compared with treatment of chronic hepatitis in adults, little is known about optimal treatment of these life-threatening conditions in children. For chronic hepatitis B and C infection, interferon-α and ribavirin have shown promise. The long-term response to these agents remains unknown; ongoing studies may answer the role of these agents in the treatment of this condition.

254. The answer is c. *(Behrman, 16/e, p. 212. McMillan, 3/e, p. 69. Rudolph, 20/e, p. 1324.)* A moribund state is characteristic of a loss of greater than 10 percent of body weight from dehydration. The other findings are characteristic of a loss of body weight of 5 percent to 9 percent when there is no hypernatremia. Additional findings at this level of dehydration can be restlessness, absent or reduced tears, weak radial pulses, and possibly, orthostatic hypotension.

255. The answer is a. *(Behrman, 16/e, pp. 212–215. McMillan, 3/e, pp. 69–71. Rudolph, 20/e, p. 1326.)* The extracellular fluid and circulating blood volumes tend to be preserved with hypernatremic dehydration at the expense of the intracellular volume. Therefore, hypotension may not be characteristic, and neither are the other signs of circulatory inadequacy that are typical of isotonic or hypotonic dehydration. Signs suggesting involvement of the central nervous system (such as irritability or lethargy) are characteristic of hypertonic dehydration. Reintroduction of a more regular diet should begin as soon as tolerated by the patient. Hypercalcemia is an infrequent finding in patients who have hypernatremic dehydration. Slow correction of this hypernatremia (over 24 to 48 hours) prevents significant fluid shifts and increased intercranial pressure.

256. The answer is b. *(Behrman, 16/e, pp. 215–218. McMillan, 3/e, pp. 71–72, 1658. Rudolph, 20/e, p. 566.)* The solution outlined in **(B)** has the actual composition of the oral rehydration solution recommended by the World Health Organization. The glucose concentrations in solutions **(C)** and **(E)** are too high and can cause osmotic diarrhea in some patients. The sodium concentrations of solutions **(D)** and **(E)** are too high for continuing use beyond the first few hours of deficit correction because hypernatremia would develop. The sodium composition of solution **(A)** is too low to replace losses and hyponatremia would develop.

257. The answer is a. *(Behrman, 16/e, pp. 37, 1109. McMillan, 3/e, pp. 642–643. Rudolph, 20/e, pp. 978–979.)* In general, mandibular teeth erupt before maxillary teeth; teeth tend to erupt in girls before boys. The first teeth to erupt usually are the mandibular central incisors at 5 to 7 months, followed by the maxillary central incisors at 6 to 8 months. Lateral incisors (mandibular then maxillary) erupt next at 7 to 11 months followed by the first molars (10 to 16 months), the cuspids (16 to 20 months), and the second molars (20 to 30 months).

258. The answer is d. *(Behrman, 16/e, pp. 1114–1116. McMillan, 3/e, pp. 651–652, 1287–1288. Rudolph, 20/e, p. 986.)* The pattern of dental disease described is diagnostic of tooth decay associated with the use of bottles that contain high concentrations of sugars, which promotes dental disease. Prevention of this disease is possible through counseling families to avoid the use of fruit juices in bottles or sweetened pacifiers.

259. The answer is d. *(Behrman, 16/e, pp. 1176–1178. McMillan, 3/e, pp. 1685–1686. Rudolph, 20/e, pp. 1032–1034.)* Recurrent abdominal pain is a common complaint occurring in at least 10 percent of school-aged children. In children older than 2 years, less than 10 percent of cases have an identifiable organic cause. Management of these children is difficult and frustrating for the physician and the family. Excessive testing and treatments are contraindicated. A thorough history and physical examination, including growth parameters, are frequently helpful in separating organic from nonorganic causes of abdominal pain. Any signs or symptoms of organic causes should be pursued. If nothing in the history or physical examination is found, as is likely in the case described, reassurance of the children and family members is indicated. Close follow-up for new or changing symptoms as well as further reassurance to the family is important.

260. The answer is a. *(Behrman, 16/e, p. 1185–1188. McMillan, 3/e, pp. 1640–1642. Rudolph, 20/e, pp. 1072–1073.)* Inguinal hernias are commonly seen in premature infants (up to 16 percent to 25 percent). Incarceration is common; elective repair is often considered prior to hospital discharge. The diagnosis is so common that rarely are diagnostic tests indicated.

261. The answer is d. *(Behrman, 16/e, pp. 1117–1118. McMillan, 3/e, pp. 655–656. Rudolph, 20/e, pp. 989–991.)* The earlier that permanent teeth are replanted the greater the rate of success, going down from 95 percent in the first 30 min to 5 percent after 2 h. The rate of success is a function of the integrity of the periodontal ligament. The teeth can be rinsed in cold water but not brushed to avoid damage to the root and periodontal ligament. Milk is a good transport medium if the child is uncooperative or for some other reason the teeth cannot be reinserted at the scene. Teeth may also be transported in the mouth of the older, cooperative patient or their parent. The immediate application of acrylic splints is needed to keep the teeth in place, so immediate dental attention is required. The need for full tetanus immunization should be evaluated.

262. The answer is b. *(Behrman, 16/e, pp. 1126–1127. McMillan, 3/e, pp. 618–619. Rudolph, 20/e, pp. 1062–1063.)* Endoscopic examination of the esophagus and stomach is a diagnostic method of determining the extent of the mucosal injury. Vomiting is to be avoided since it would expose the mucosal surfaces to the caustic agent a second time. The child can be given small amounts of milk or water, but large amounts, which might cause vomiting, are unwise. Neutralization of the caustic can result in an exothermic reaction and produce a thermal burn. The use of steroids after endoscopy in second-degree chemical burns of the esophagus has been effective in diminishing the inflammatory response in some patients. Optimal treatment is still controversial and requires expert consultation or review of the most current literature. Charcoal, however, does not absorb the alkaline agent in drain cleaner.

263. The answer is c. *(Behrman, 16/e, pp. 2161–2162, 2167. McMillan, 3/e, pp. 618–619. Rudolph, 20/e, pp. 815–816.)* The absorption of toxins from the gastrointestinal tract is diminished by the use of activated charcoal administered during the first few hours after the ingestion in the minimum dose of 1 g per kilogram of body weight or 5 to 10 times the quantity of the ingested material. Activated charcoal exerts its effect by adsorbing particles of toxin on its surface. Compounds not adsorbed include alcohols, acids, ferrous sulfate, strong bases, cyanide, lithium, and potassium. For drugs with an enterohepatic circulation (e.g., phenobarbital and tricyclic antidepressants), or those with prolonged absorption (e.g., sustained-release theophylline), the use of multiple-dose activated charcoal can be effective in decreasing the half-life and increasing the total body clearance of the toxic substance.

264–268. The answers are 264–b,d; 265–b; 266–e; 267–c,e; 268–c. *(Behrman, 16/e, pp. 1183–1184. McMillan, 3/e, pp. 647, 696, 1644. Rudolph, 20/e, pp. 962, 1109–1110.)* All the disorders listed have gastrointestinal polyposis. Peutz-Jeghers syndrome, which is inherited as an autosomal dominant trait, is characterized by the presence of hamartomatous polyps, especially in the small intestine but also occasionally in the stomach and colon. The most striking extraintestinal manifestation of this disorder is lip or buccal pigmentation, which usually develops during infancy. Peutz-Jeghers polyposis rarely leads to carcinoma.

Gardner's syndrome, on the other hand, is characterized by adenomatous polyps that frequently undergo malignant degeneration. This autosomal dominant disorder occurs mainly in the colon but can also involve the small intestine. In affected children under the age of 10 years, the condition can appear first as a fibromatous mass or epidermoid cyst involving skin or soft tissue, especially of the mandible.

Isolated juvenile polyps are very common (3 percent to 4 percent of the population) and occur as a benign, nonheritable condition typically associated with pedunculated inflammatory polyps that usually appear within 25 cm of the anus. Familial polyposis of the colon, in contrast, is a dominantly inherited condition causing large numbers of juvenile polyps to appear in the intestine, possibly in the spectrum of diseases including Gardner's syndrome. Although children with juvenile polyposis of the colon can have other congenital anomalies and there is a risk of malignant degeneration, children with juvenile polyps usually do not have these problems.

Hemangiomas of the intestine are rare but benign lesions that can cause severe, even fatal, painless hemorrhage from the intestines. About 50 percent of patients will have associated cutaneous hemangiomas; a few will have a family history. Relationship to colon cancer is questionable.

269–274. The answers are 269–d, 270–c, 271–b, 272–c, 273–b, 274–c. *(Behrman, 16/e, pp. 155–156, 215–218, McMillan, 3/e, pp. 476, 1656–1664.)* It is important to know the composition of fluids that can be used in infant feedings, particularly in infants with diarrhea, which may be exacerbated by inappropriate choices. Cola has over three times the carbohydrate concentration of cow's milk, 16.6 g/dL compared with 4.9 g/dL, and over twice the carbohydrate concentration of human milk, 7 g/dl, but has almost the same caloric density as both milks—about 670 cal/L. Almost all the calories of cola come from carbohydrate, making it (as well as apple juice) inadequate as a major dietary component for infants or children. Apple juice and cola provide a surprisingly large amount of calories (particularly for those who wish to limit caloric consumption) and can also present an unreasonably large load for absorption to the gastrointestinal tract of patients prone to diarrhea. It can increase water loss in the stools by an osmotic effect. The carbohydrate concentration of oral rehydration solution (WHO) is 2% glucose, which is enough to help fluid absorption in cotransport with sodium while avoiding excess. All the solutions have adequate amounts of potassium, but the fruit juices have almost no sodium.

This combination of factors makes an oral rehydration solution or human milk more appropriate than the other solutions for treating acute diarrhea. The WHO rehydration solution has a higher concentration of sodium than do the commercially available oral rehydration solutions commonly used in the United States. The WHO solution is often used for treating cholera, in which the stools contain much more NaCl than in the ordinary diarrheal stool.

275–278. The answers are 275–g, 276–e, 277–b, 278–d. (*Behrman, 16/e, pp. 167, 404–405, 1157–1159, 1165–1167, 1214–1216, 1315–1327, 1743. McMillan, 3/e, pp. 1242–1254, 1694–1697, 1957–1958, 1750, 2055, 2174–2175. Rudolph, 20/e, pp. 98–100, 494, 965, 1103, 1081–1082, 1085–1087, 1640–1641, 1889–1890, 1997, 2026–2027.*) Reye's syndrome is becoming increasingly rare. Its hallmarks are acute encephalopathy and fatty degeneration of the liver. The association of this disease with aspirin use in children having recently suffered a bout with influenza or varicella has resulted in a dramatic decrease in aspirin use in children. No tests are diagnostic of this condition, although elevated liver function studies and serum ammonia levels are helpful. Diagnosis of this condition is dependent on a high index of suspicion. Treatment is supportive.

Cystic fibrosis is a multisystem disease primarily affecting the lungs and the intestines. Respiratory symptoms upon presentation include cough with frequent pneumonias. Intestinal symptoms include large, bulky, foul-smelling stools in the failure-to-thrive infant. It is most common in white children and far less common in Hispanics and blacks. The diagnosis is made with the sweat test and chromosomal analysis.

Colic is a frustrating condition for the child, the parents, and the physician. It commonly occurs before the age of 3 months and is of unknown etiology. The child has the sudden onset of crying for several hours, the abdomen is tense and distended, the legs are drawn up to the abdomen, and the child frequently passes gas. Many theories have been forwarded as to the cause, including swallowed air, milk intolerance, and maternal dietary changes. After a careful history and physical examination reveals no other likely pathology, reassurance to the parents is indicated. A variety of measures such as feeding the child in the upright position (avoiding air swallowing), frequent burping, gentle rocking, assistance in passing stools or flatus, and other measures are commonly tried with a variable response.

A permanent sensitivity to dietary gluten (commonly found in wheat, rye, oats, and barley) results in small-bowel mucosal damage in gluten's presence. Affected children usually present between 1 to 2 years of age with diarrhea, but can also present with failure to thrive (frequently with food avoidance) or vomiting. Clinically, children can have abdominal distention and pallor. Laboratory tests can reveal anemia and hypoproteinemia.

Small-bowel biopsy is the gold standard for diagnosis. A lifelong, gluten-free diet is curative.

Behçet's syndrome is a vasculitis of small- or medium-sized arteries and veins. Classically, this causes a nondestructive arthritis in multiple joints, especially large joints such as knees. Associated symptoms include fever, erythema nodosum, aphthous stomatitis, uveitis, and central nervous system abnormalities ranging from trivial complaints to pseudotumor cerebri.

Wolman's syndrome is a lysosomal acid lipase deficiency. It presents in infancy with hepatosplenomegaly, diarrhea and vomiting, failure to thrive, icterus, and malabsorption. A KUB shows calcification of the adrenal gland. There is no treatment known for this condition.

Short-gut syndrome is caused by perinatal events including volvulus, gastroschisis, small bowel atresia, necrotizing enterocolitis, meconium ileus, Crohn's disease, and trauma. Nutrient malabsorption can occur. High-quality oral feeds, potentially with parenteral nutrition, can be required.

THE URINARY TRACT

Questions

DIRECTIONS: Each item below contains a question or incomplete statement followed by suggested responses. Select the **one best** response to each question.

279. The presence of drug-induced nephrotic syndrome should be most highly suspected in a proteinuric patient who has received which of the following drugs?

a. tetracycline
b. streptomycin
c. trimethadione
d. diazepam
e. chlorambucil

280. The delivery of a newborn boy is remarkable for oligohydramnios. The infant is noted to have a remarkably thin, wrinkled abdominal wall and undescended testes, club feet, and to be in respiratory distress. The most likely diagnosis to explain these findings is

a. surfactant deficiency
b. Turner's syndrome
c. prune-belly syndrome
d. hermaphrodite
e. congenital adrenal hyperplasia

281. A 7-year-old boy suffers multiple injuries as a result of blunt abdominal trauma. Which of the following statements concerning the proper assessment and treatment of the injuries is true?

a. most renal injuries require operative intervention
b. major vascular injuries require rapid surgical intervention
c. rupture of a full bladder is highly unlikely
d. the renal capsule surrounding the kidney precludes the need for surgical exploration and most cases of traumatic hematocele
e. visible blood in the urine following trauma nearly always indicates significant renal damage

282. A 1-year-old child presents with failure to thrive, frequent large voids of dilute urine, excessive thirst, and three episodes of dehydration not associated with vomiting or diarrhea. Over the years, other family members reportedly have had similar histories. The likely diagnosis is

a.   water intoxication
b.   diabetes mellitus
c.   diabetes insipidus
d.   child abuse
e.   nephrotic syndrome

283. Which of the following drugs is LEAST likely to be nephrotoxic?

a.   penicillamine
b.   lithium
c.   outdated tetracycline
d.   nonsteroidal anti-inflammatory drugs (NSAIDs)
e.   sulfonamide antibiotics

284. An exogenous substance that is used to measure glomerular filtration rate should be

a.   physiologically active
b.   capable of binding with plasma proteins
c.   freely filterable at the glomerulus
d.   secreted by the renal tubule
e.   reabsorbed by the renal tubule

285. After a urinary tract infection, a 1-year-old is diagnosed with grade 2 vesicourethral reflux. Which of the following is an appropriate treatment option?

a.   low dose daily antibiotics
b.   immediate surgical reimplantation of the ureters
c.   weekly urinalyses and culture
d.   diet low in protein
e.   early toilet training

Items 286–287

286. Physical examination of a baby boy shortly after birth reveals a large bladder and palpable kidneys. A voiding cystourethrogram performed on the baby demonstrates an area of obstruction and proximal dilatation of the urethra, ureters, and kidney. He appears to be otherwise normal. Which of the following is the likely diagnosis?

a. ureteropelvic junction obstruction
b. posterior urethral valve
c. prune-belly syndrome
d. duplication of the collecting system
e. horseshoe kidney

287. Despite vigorous medical and surgical efforts, this child with a severe obstructive uropathy has an 80 percent reduction of glomerular filtration rate and elevated levels of blood (BUN) urea nitrogen and creatinine. He is in chronic renal failure. He may eventually exhibit which of the following?

a. polycythemia
b. rickets
c. frequent episodes of hypoglycemia
d. early onset of puberty
e. metabolic alkalosis

288. Funduscopic examination of a 13-year-old girl shows general and focal arteriolar narrowing. A hemorrhage is observed in the left retina, and sclerosis is present. Her blood pressure is 180/110 mm Hg. This girl would be likely to exhibit which of the following symptoms or signs.

a. multiple cranial nerve palsy
b. headache
c. hyporeflexia
d. increased urine output
e. right ventricular hypertrophy

289. A 2-year-old boy with undescended testes is referred to a urologist. Surgical correction will probably eliminate the risk of

a. testicular malignancy
b. decreased sperm count
c. torsion of testes
d. urinary tract infection
e. epididymitis

290. An *Escherichia coli* colony count of $2000/mm^3$ would be definite evidence of a urinary tract infection if the sampled urine

a. has a specific gravity of 1.008
b. is from a clean catch urine in an 8-year-old uncircumcised boy
c. is from an ileal-loop bag
d. is from a suprapubic tap
e. is the first morning sample

291. A 6-year-old black boy has brown urine and healing impetigo lesions. He presents with hypertension, dyspnea, periorbital edema, and hepatomegaly. The most likely cause of his problem is

a. IgA nephropathy
b. post-streptococcal glomerulonephritis
c. idiopathic hypercalciuria
d. pyelonephritis
e. sexually transmitted disease

292. A 2-year-old boy develops bloody diarrhea shortly after eating in a fast-food restaurant. A few days later, he develops pallor and lethargy; his face looks swollen and his mother reports that he has been urinating very little. Laboratory evaluation reveals low hematocrit and platelet count and positive blood and protein in the urine. Which of the following diagnoses is likely to explain these symptoms?

a. Henoch-Schönlein purpura
b. IgA nephropathy
c. intussusception
d. Meckel's diverticulum
e. hemolytic-uremic syndrome

293. A 6-year-old girl is brought to the emergency room because her urine is red. She has been healthy and asymptomatic otherwise. Which of the following conditions would result in a positive dipstick for heme?

a. ingestion of blackberries
b. ingestion of beets
c. phenolphthalein catharsis
d. presence of myoglobin
e. ingestion of Kool-Aid

294. The pictured photomicrograph of a urine specimen from a 7-year-old child is LEAST likely to support a diagnosis of

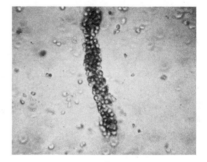

a. systemic lupus erythematosus
b. acute poststreptococcal glomerulonephritis
c. Berger's disease
d. membranous glomerulopathy
e. mesangiocapillary glomerulonephritis

295. A 5-year-old boy comes to the emergency department at midnight with a complaint of severe scrotal pain since 7 P.M. There is no history of trauma. Your first step is to

a. order a surgical consult immediately
b. order a radioisotope scan as an emergency
c. order a urinalysis and Gram's stain for bacteria
d. arrange for an ultrasound examination
e. order a Doppler examination

296. During the first year of an infant's life, which of the following remains essentially unchanged?

a. glomerular filtration rate
b. nephron number
c. renal blood flow
d. tubular reabsorptive capacity
e. ability to concentrate urine

297. A 7-year-old boy has crampy abdominal pain and a rash mainly on the back of his legs and buttocks as well as on the extensor surfaces of his forearms. Laboratory analysis reveals proteinuria and microhematuria. He is most likely to be affected by

a. systemic lupus erythematosus
b. anaphylactoid purpura
c. post-streptococcal glomerulonephritis
d. Takayasu arteritis
e. dermatomyositis

298. A 16-year-old boy complains of several months of swelling but no pain just above his left testicle. He is sexually active but states that he uses condoms. On physical examination, he has a mass along the spermatic cord that feels like a "bag of worms." Which of the following is appropriate for this condition?

a. Doppler flow study of testes
b. radionuclide scan of testes
c. urinalysis and culture
d. ceftriaxone intramuscularly and doxycycline orally
e. reassurance and education only at this time

299. A 3-day-old infant's left side of the scrotum is larger than the right. Palpation reveals a tense, fluid-filled area surrounding the right testicle. The scrotum transilluminates well and the amount of fluid does not vary with mild pressure. The appropriate approach to this condition is to

a. request a surgical consultation
b. begin furosemide orally
c. administer prophylactic antibiotics
d. observe only
e. perform a chromosome determination

300. A 2-year-old patient has microscopic and occasionally gross hematuria. His father has hearing loss and end-stage renal disease. The most likely cause of this child's hematuria is

a. Alport's syndrome
b. Berger's nephropathy (IgA nephropathy)
c. idiopathic hypercalciuria
d. membranous glomerulopathy
e. Goodpasture's syndrome

301. Which of the following statements concerning nocturnal enuresis is correct?

a. the condition is three times more common in girls than boys
b. most patients with enuresis have a psychiatric illness as the cause
c. spontaneous cure rates are high regardless of therapy
d. family history of enuresis is uncommon
e. short courses of desmopressin acetate (DDAVP) lead to permanent cure in 25 percent of cases

302. A 21-year-old woman presents to the emergency room in active labor. She has had no prenatal care but her last menstrual period was approximately 9 months prior. Her membranes are artificially ruptured, yielding no amniotic fluid. She delivers an 1800-g term infant who develops significant respiratory distress immediately at birth. The first chest radiograph on this infant demonstrates hypoplastic lungs. Which of the following is an appropriate next step for this infant?

a. cardiac catheterization
b. renal ultrasound
c. MRI of the brain
d. liver and spleen scan
e. upper GI

DIRECTIONS: Each group of questions below consists of lettered options followed by numbered items. For each numbered item, select the appropriate lettered option(s). Each lettered option may be used once, more than once, or not at all. **Choose exactly the number of options indicated following each item.**

Items 303–306

For each condition listed below, match the category to which it belongs.

a. nephrotic syndrome
b. renal tubular acidosis
c. Bartter's syndrome
d. acute glomerulonephritis
e. IgA nephropathy (Berger's nephropathy)
f. idiopathic hypercalciuria

303. Serum protein of 1.5 g/dL
(SELECT 1 DISORDER)

304. Hypertension as a typical complication
(SELECT 1 DISORDER)

305. Elevated levels of cholesterol and triglycerides
(SELECT 1 DISORDER)

306. Growth failure and hypokalemia
(SELECT 1 DISORDER)

THE URINARY TRACT

Answers

279. The answer is c. *(Behrman, 16/e, pp. 1592–1596. McMillan, 3/e, pp. 590–591.)* Drug-related nephrotic syndrome has been described in connection with the use of trimethadione, penicillamine, tolbutamide, and certain heavy metals. Nephrosis can develop in conjunction with malignancy.

280. The answer is c. *(Behrman, 16/e, pp. 1635–1637. McMillan, 3/e, pp. 341–342, 1558–1559. Rudolph, 20/e, pp. 215–216, 1399–1400.)* Prune-belly syndrome, a malformation that occurs mostly in males, is characterized by a lax, wrinkled abdominal wall, a dilated urinary tract, and intraabdominal testes. There are additional urinary tract abnormalities including significant renal dysfunction or dysplasia. Oligohydramnios and commonly associated pulmonary complications, such as pulmonary hypoplasia and pneumothorax, are seen frequently. Congenital hip dislocation, club feet, and intestinal malrotation with possible secondary volvulus can occur. There does not appear to be a genetic predisposition to prune-belly syndrome.

281. The answer is b. *(Behrman, 16/e, pp. 1654–1655. McMillan, 3/e, p. 2214. Rudolph, 20/e, pp. 1048–1049.)* Most injuries to the kidney are mild and do not require surgery but rather, close observation. Identification of those with the serious injury requiring surgery can be difficult. The CT scan or intravenous pyelogram are helpful to identify serious injury (i.e., those with major vascular injury requiring rapid surgical intervention or those with traumatic hydroceles). Because it is an abdominal organ in children, the bladder, especially when full, is often ruptured by blunt trauma and lower abdominal wounds. Although small bladder tears can be treated conservatively by catheter drainage, surgical exploration is likely to be needed. Extensive urethral injuries can require surgical drainage of periurethral hematoma, primary surgical repair, or even urinary diversion procedures. Most ureteral injuries require prompt surgical intervention, although such injuries are rare because of the protected position of the ureter. A retrograde cystourethrogram and intravenous urography can be helpful, especially with pelvic fracture or suspected renal trauma.

282. The answer is c. *(Behrman, 16/e, pp. 1600–1601. McMillan, 3/e, pp. 1621–1622, 1789. Rudolph, 20/e, pp. 1382–1383.)* Nephrogenic diabetes insipidus is a hereditary congenital disorder in which the urine is hypotonic and produced in large volumes because the kidneys fail to respond to antidiuretic hormone. Most North American patients thus involved are descendants of Ulster Scots who came to Nova Scotia in 1761 on the ship Hopewell. Males are primarily affected, apparently through an X-linked recessive modal, though there can be a variable expression in heterozygous females. The defect is unknown, but the disorder is felt to result from primary unresponsiveness of the distal tubule and collecting duct to vasopressin. Although the condition is present at birth, the diagnosis is often not made until several months later, when excessive thirst, frequent voiding of large volumes of dilute urine, dehydration, and failure to thrive become obvious. Maintenance of adequate fluid intake and diet and use of saluretic drugs are the bases of therapy for this incurable disease. Water intoxication would not present with episodes of dehydration; diabetes mellitus rarely presents with a protracted course in such a young child (it is usually a more acute illness and often with vomiting). Child abuse would be unlikely, especially with a family history as noted. Nephrotic syndrome would be expected to present with other signs such as edema, proteinuria, and other symptoms.

283. The answer is e. *(Behrman, 16/e, pp. 1603–1604. McMillan, 3/e, pp. 1613, 2202. Rudolph, 20/e, pp. 509, 1376, 1380–1381.)* Many commonly used medications, chemicals, and diagnostic agents are potentially nephrotoxic. The mechanisms of actions of these agents is through acute tubular necrosis, alteration of renal blood flow, intratubular obstruction, or allergic reactions within the kidney itself. Many of these toxic effects are reduced or eliminated with removal of the offending agent. Nephrotic syndrome is associated with penicillamine; lithium can cause renal tubular acidosis and nephrogenic diabetes insipidus; outdated tetracycline causes Fanconi's syndrome; and NSAIDs can cause nephrotic syndrome or interstitial nephritis. In the past, sulfonamide agents had been insoluble, resulting in renal disease; newer agents do not have this toxicity.

284. The answer is c. *(Behrman, 16/e, pp. 1574–1575. McMillan, 3/e, p. 73.)* If an exogenous substance is capable of being metabolized, bound by plasma proteins, or secreted or reabsorbed by the renal tubule, it will not measure glomerular function adequately.

285. The answer is a. *(Behrman, 16/e, pp. 1625–1629. McMillan, 3/e, pp. 1548–1549. Rudolph, 20/e, pp. 1398–1399.)* In children, primary reflux of urine into the ureter and kidney is more common. The higher the reflux into the renal system, especially if the renal pelvis is dilated, the more likely it is for renal damage to occur. Low grade lesions (grade 1 and grade 2) are conservatively managed with close watching, daily low dose antibiotics, and urinalyses and cultures every 3 to 4 months. Higher grade lesions (grade 4 and grade 5) often are treated with surgical reimplantation of a ureter. Those lesions in between these two extremes are treatment dilemmas.

286. The answer is b. *(Behrman, 16/e, pp. 1636–1637. McMillan, 3/e, pp. 1549–1551. Rudolph, 20/e, pp. 1397–1398.)* The constellation of findings described points to posterior urethral valves. The clinical picture may range from that described in the question to severe renal obstruction with renal failure and pulmonary hypoplasia. Urinary tract infections are common complications in older children, and sepsis can occasionally be the presenting sign in afflicted newborns. Despite early recognition and correction of the obstruction, the prognosis for normal renal function is guarded. Prenatal diagnosis is often accomplished secondary to ultrasound diagnosis.

287. The answer is b. *(Behrman, 16/e, pp. 1609–1611. McMillan, 3/e, pp. 1568–1572. Rudolph, 20/e, pp. 1309–1310, 1340–1347, 1355–1358.)* Renal osteodystrophy, which occurs in chronic renal failure, is a designation that encompasses osteitis fibrosa cystica, caused by secondary hyperparathyroidism, and rickets, or osteomalacia, caused by deficiency of $1,25(OH)_2D_3$; they can occur together. Growth retardation, rather than precocious puberty, occurs in chronic real failure due to: malnutrition (poor appetite, low somatomedin C level), renal osteodystrophy, excessive urinary loss of water and sodium, metabolic acidosis, and anemia. Bone age is lower than chronologic age. Neurodevelopmental problems occur, especially when uremia develops during early infancy. Brain growth is subnormal and gross motor and developmental delays occur. In untreated children, progressive encephalopathy ensues. Normocytic, normochromic anemia is seen in advanced chronic renal failure, mainly as a result of a relative deficiency of erythropoietin; its other causes include shortened life span of red blood cells in uremic patients, gastrointestinal blood loss caused by abnormal platelet function, iatrogenic blood loss during hemodialysis and from frequent blood sampling, folic acid deficiency, dialysis-related aluminum toxicity, and poor appetite. Glucose intolerance results from peripheral resistance to endogenous insulin. Elevated glucagon and growth hormone levels may be contributing factors.

288. The answer is b. *(Behrman, 16/e, pp. 1450–1455. McMillan, 3/e, pp. 1433–1434. Rudolph, 20/e, p. 1547.)* Hypertension is usually asymptomatic but with marked hypertension, children can develop headache, dizziness, visual disturbances, irritability, and nocturnal wakening. Hypertensive encephalopathy can be preceded or accompanied by vomiting, hyperreflexia, ataxia, and focal or generalized seizures. Facial nerve palsy can be the sole manifestation of severe hypertension. Isolated left ventricular hypertrophy, decreased urine output, and abdominal bruits may be possible. When marked fundal changes are present or when there are signs of vascular compromise, emergency treatment of the accompanying hypertension is warranted. Such hypertensive persons require immediate hospitalization for diagnosis and therapy.

289. The answer is c. *(Behrman, 16/e, pp. 1650–1651. McMillan, 3/e, pp. 1555–1556. Rudolph, 20/e, pp. 1404–1405.)* At 1 year of age, 0.7 percent of boys born at term still have cryptorchidism. In adults with cryptorchidism, the risk of testicular malignancy is much higher than in unaffected men. Orchiopexy does not eliminate this risk, but repositioning the testes makes them accessible for periodic examinations. Whether the testes are brought into the scrotum or not, the sperm count can be reduced. The failure of the testes to develop, and their subsequent atrophy, can be detected by 6 months of age. Torsion of the testis is a potential risk because of the excessive mobility of the undescended testis. Orchiopexy helps to eliminate this problem.

290. The answer is d. *(Behrman, 16/e, pp. 1622–1623. McMillan, 3/e, pp. 420–421. Rudolph, 20/e, p. 1332.)* No bacteria at all should grow in a properly obtained urine sample from a suprapubic tap or from retrograde catheterization of the upper urinary tract unless infection is present. Thus, any bacterial growth at all from a properly obtained suprapubic tap is significant. Ileal-loop bags are usually contaminated. Colony counts greater than 10^5 on properly obtained clean-catch urines are significant. Clean-catch urines in an uncircumcised male who cannot retract the foreskin are suspect.

291. The answer is b. (*Behrman, 16/e, pp. 1579–1582, 1587. McMillan, 3/e, pp. 1583–1586. Rudolph, 20/e, pp. 1353–1354.*) Acute post-streptococcal glomerulonephritis follows a skin or throat infection with certain nephritogenic strains of group A β-hemolytic streptococci. Hematuria often colors the urine dark, and decreased urinary output can result in circulatory congestion from volume overload with pulmonary edema, periorbital edema, tachycardia, and hepatomegaly. This can be avoided by fluid restriction. Acute hypertension is common and can be associated with headache, vomiting, and encephalopathy with seizures. Pyelonephritis and sexually transmitted diseases can cause bloody urine, but rarely the other symptoms of impetigo as described in the question.

IgA nephropathy is rare in black children and rarely presents with hypertension. Idiopathic hypercalciuria can present with blood and renal stones, but the other findings are distinctly unusual.

292. The answer is e. (*Behrman, 16/e, pp. 1586–1587. McMillan, 3/e, pp. 2204–2206. Rudolph, 20/e, pp. 1361–1362.*) Hemolytic uremic syndrome is characterized by an acute microangiopathic hemolytic anemia, thrombocytopenia from increased platelet utilization, and renal insufficiency from vascular endothelial injury and local fibrin deposition. Ischemic changes result in renal cortical necrosis and damage to other organs such as colon, liver, heart, brain, and adrenal. Laboratory findings associated with hemolytic uremic syndrome include low hemoglobin level, decreased platelet count, hypoalbuminemia, and evidence of hemolysis on peripheral smear (burr cells, helmet cells, schistocytes). Urinalysis reveals hematuria and proteinuria. A marked reduction of renal function leads to oliguria and rising levels of blood urea nitrogen (BUN) and creatinine. Gastrointestinal bleeding and obstruction, ascites, and central nervous system findings such as somnolence, convulsions, and coma can occur. In the past decade, infection by the verotoxin-producing *Escherichia coli* 0157:H7 has been implicated as a cause of hemolytic uremic syndrome. This organism is epizootic in cattle. Outbreaks associated with undercooked contaminated hamburgers have been reported in several states. Roast beef, cow's milk, and fresh apple cider have been implicated as well. The Coombs' test is not positive in this type of hemolytic anemia.

293. The answer is d. *(Behrman, 16/e, p. 1577. Rudolph, 20/e, p. 1332.)* A number of pH-dependent substances can impart a red color to urine. Use of phenolphthalein, a cathartic agent, or phenindione, an anticoagulant, can cause red urine; ingestion of blackberries or beets also can lead to red coloration ("beeturia"). None of these choices, however, would cause the heme test to be positive. Myoglobin, on the other hand, does test positive for heme. It is the only choice that can test positive for heme. Hematuria should be confirmed by dipstick testing as well as by microscopic examination of urinary sediment.

294. The answer is d. *(McMillan, 3/e, pp. 1583 1587, 1591, 1596. Rudolph, 20/e, pp. 1333, 1353–1351, 1359–1361, 1361–1365.)* The figure accompanying the question depicts a red blood cell cast characteristically found in the urine of patients with glomerular disease. Important exceptions include the minimal lesion form of the nephrotic syndrome and membranous glomerulopathy. In these, the urine contains large amounts of protein and hyaline casts but few red blood cells.

295. The answer is a. *(McMillan, 3/e, pp. 1556–1557. Rudolph, 20/e, p. 1404.)* The majority of all cases of acute scrotal pain and swelling in boys under 6 years of age are caused by testicular torsion. If surgical exploration occurs within 4 to 6 hours, the testes can be saved 90 percent of the time. Too often, delay caused by scheduling of various imaging modalities and laboratory tests results in an unsalvageable gonad.

296. The answer is b. *(McMillan, 3/e, pp. 336–340. Rudolph, 20/e, pp. 1316–1319.)* The kidneys of a newborn infant already contain their full complement of nephrons. Glomerular filtration rate and renal plasma flow steadily increase to close to normal adult values (corrected for surface area) by the end of the first year of life. Infants have a relatively low rate of sodium reabsorption, which increases proportionally as body weight increases. The secretion of substances such as para-aminohippuric acid increases during the first year of life, as does the infant's ability to concentrate the urine.

297. The answer is b. *(Behrman, 16/e, pp. 728–729. McMillan, 3/e, pp. 2176–2179. Rudolph, 20/e, pp. 909–911, 1240–1241, 1359.)* The rash of anaphylactoid purpura most often involves extensor surfaces of the extremities; the face, soles, palms, and trunk are less often affected. Other significant symptoms include edema, arthralgia or arthritis, colicky abdominal pain with GI bleeding, acute scrotal pain, and renal abnormalities ranging from microscopic hematuria to renal failure. Both systemic lupus erythematosus and dermatomyositis are often accompanied by typical facial rashes (butterfly and heliotrope, respectively). People who have Takayasu arteritis usually do not present with a rash. The scarlatiniform rash characteristic of streptococcal infections generally does not coincide with the development of post-streptococcal nephritis; impetiginous lesions, however, may still be present.

298. The answer is e. *(Behrman, 16/e, p. 1653. McMillan, 3/e, p. 1558. Rudolph, 20/e, p. 59.)* Varicocele, a common condition seen after 10 years of age, occurs in about 15 percent of adult males. It results from the dilatation of the pampiniform venous plexus (usually on the left side) due to valvular incompetence of the spermatic vein. Reduced sperm counts are possible with this condition; surgery may ultimately be indicated for infertility problems. Typically, these lesions are not painful but can become tender with strenuous exercise. Its typical bag of worms appearance on palpation makes its diagnosis apparent in most cases. For a 16-year-old boy, reassurance and education seem appropriate.

299. The answer is d. *(Behrman, 16/e, p. 1653. McMillan, 3/e, pp. 1557–1558, 1640–1641. Rudolph, 20/e, pp. 1072–1073, 1403–1404.)* The description is that of a hydrocele, an accumulation of fluid in the tunica vaginalis. Small hydroceles usually resolve spontaneously in the first year of life. Larger ones or those that have a variable fluid level with time will likely need surgical repair.

300. The answer is a. *(Behrman, 16/e, p. 1580. McMillan, 3/e, pp. 1599–1601. Rudolph, 20/e, pp. 1371–1372.)* The most common type of hereditary nephritis is Alport's syndrome. Clinically, patients present with asymptomatic microscopic hematuria, but gross hematuria is also possible. Hearing loss, eventually leading to deafness, is associated with Alport's syndrome in 30 percent to 75 percent of cases. End-stage renal disease is common by the second or third decades of life. This syndrome is thought to be an X-linked dominant disorder, which explains the more severe course in males.

301. The answer is c. *(Behrman, 16/e, pp. 72–73. McMillan, 3/e, pp. 1559–1600. Rudolph, 20/e, pp. 1336–1337.)* Nocturnal enuresis is involuntary voiding at night at an age when control of micturition is expected. It is common in children under the age of 5 years (approximately 20 percent), resolving in approximately 15 percent of these cases per year thereafter. A careful history and physical examination will usually identify any potential organic causes. In most cases, no etiology is found. A family history is common. Minimal laboratory testing beyond screening urinalysis is indicated. The condition is more common in boys than in girls. Therapy is aimed at reassurance to the parents that the condition is self-limited, avoidance of punitive measures, and consideration of purchasing a bed-wetting alarm. Spontaneous cure rates are high regardless of therapy. Short courses of DDAVP lead to control in 60 percent to 75 percent of cases while the patient takes the medication, but frequently the episodes return when the medication is stopped.

302. The answer is b. *(Behrman, 16/e, p. 461. McMillan, 3/e, p. 1336. Rudolph, 20/e, pp. 1393–1396.)* Oligohydramnios can cause a number of serious problems in the infant, including constraint deformities (such as clubfoot) and pulmonary hypoplasia. These infants have usually experienced intrauterine growth retardation and frequently have an associated serious renal abnormality. Ultrasound of the kidneys is important to rule out renal involvement as a cause of the oligohydramnios.

303–306. The answers are 303–a, 304–d, 305–a, 306–c. *(Behrman, 16/e, pp. 1577–1578, 1592–1596, 1601–1602. McMillan, 3/e, pp. 1590–1599, 1624–1625. Rudolph, 20/e, pp. 1351–1354, 1366–1367, 1383–1384.)* Elevated levels of cholesterol and triglycerides are common in nephrotic syndrome because of generalized protein synthesis in the liver (including lipoproteins) and because of a decrease in lipid metabolism due to reduced plasma lipoprotein lipase levels. In the nephrotic syndrome, albumin is lost in the urine and, despite increased hepatic synthesis, serum levels drop. The upper limit of protein excretion in healthy children is 0.15g/24 h. In nephrotic syndrome, proteinuria can exceed 2.0g/24 h. When the level drops low enough, the oncotic pressure of the plasma becomes too low to balance the hydrostatic pressure. Plasma volume, therefore, decreases as edema occurs. Endocrine and renal mechanisms then partially compensate by retaining water and salt. Careful monitoring and restriction of water and salt intake are not usually required. With acute glomerulo-nephritis, on the other hand, oliguria frequently occurs as a direct consequence of the disease process itself, and on occasion, it can be profound with virtual anuria for several days. During this period of time, it is vital to monitor and restrict fluid intake lest massive edema, hypervolemia, and even pulmonary edema and death occur. Hypertension commonly accompanies glomerulonephritis, but only occasionally accompanies nephrotic syndrome. Diuretics are sometimes used in both nephrotic syndrome and glomeralonephritis with temporary effect, but are not curative. A combination of albumin infusions followed by a diuretic also has been used to temporarily decrease the edema in patients with nephrotic syndrome. Because both illnesses are usually self-limited, temporary measures are important.

Bartter's syndrome (also known as juxtaglomerular hyperplasia) causes hypokalemia, alkalosis, hyperaldosteronism, normotension, and hyper-reninemia. It may be inherited as an autosomal recessive trait. Clinical presentations occurring frequently between 6 to 12 months of age include failure to thrive with constipation, weakness, vomiting, polyuria, and poly-dipsia. Treatment is aimed at returning the potassium level to normal.

THE NEUROMUSCULAR SYSTEM

Questions

DIRECTIONS: Each item below contains a question or incomplete statement followed by suggested responses. Select the **one best** response to each question.

307. Among the developmental abnormalities and deviations of early childhood, the one most amenable to early intervention is

a. autism
b. mental retardation of unknown cause
c. psychomotor retardation
d. developmental language disorder
e. trisomy 21

308. A 4-year-old child falls from the back of a three-wheeled vehicle, hitting his head. He experiences no loss of consciousness. In the emergency room, he is alert and oriented without focal findings on examination. He has blood behind his left tympanic membrane. CT scan of the skull is likely to show

a. subdural hematoma
b. epidural hematoma
c. intraventricular hemorrhage
d. basilar skull fracture
e. hydrocephalus

309. The examination of a newborn's back reveals a quarter-size "lump" of soft tissue overlying the lower spine. Evaluation with ultrasound of this lesion may demonstrate

a. Ebstein pearl
b. mongolian spot
c. cephalohematoma
d. omphalocele
e. occult spina bifida

310. Which of the following aminoacidopathies can be associated with acute infantile hemiplegia?

a. phenylketonuria
b. homocystinuria
c. cystathioninuria
d. maple syrup urine disease
e. histidinemia

311. The safest way to avoid a traumatic lumbar puncture in an infant is to

a. quickly push the needle in all the way until a pop is felt
b. push the needle in until resistance is felt and then withdraw the stylet
c. use a needle without a stylet
d. twirl the needle repeatedly
e. advance the needle by small increments and remove the stylet after each advance to see if CSF comes out

312. A 4-year-old child is observed to hold his eyelids open with his fingers and to close one eye periodically, especially in the evening. He has some trouble swallowing his food. He usually appears sad, although he laughs often enough. He can throw a ball, and he runs well. Which of the following is likely to result in the diagnosis?

a. muscle biopsy
b. creatine phosphokinase (CPK)
c. effect of endrophonium on eyelids
d. chest x-ray
e. antinuclear antibodies (ANAs)

313. A 3-year-old child is unconscious with symmetrically small pupils. These findings may be found in which of the following?

a. pontine hemorrhage
b. phenylephrine overdose
c. trauma with resultant third nerve palsy
d. atropine-induced coma
e. cyclopentolate exposure

314. A previously healthy 7-year-old child suddenly complains of a headache and falls to the floor. When examined in the emergency room, he is lethargic and has a left central facial weakness and left hemiparesis with conjugate ocular deviation to the right. The most likely diagnosis is

a. hemiplegic migraine
b. supratentorial tumor
c. Todd's paralysis
d. acute subdural hematoma
e. acute infantile hemiplegia

315. The absence of hexosaminidase A activity in white blood cells confirms the diagnosis of which of the following lipidoses?

a. Niemann-Pick disease
b. infantile Gaucher's disease
c. Tay-Sachs disease
d. Krabbe's disease
e. Fabry's disease

316. Children who have myotonic dystrophy commonly exhibit which of the following?

a. hirsutism
b. seizure activity
c. severe proximal muscle weakness
d. ptosis
e. enlarged gonads

317. Characteristics of childhood migraine typically include which of the following?

a. strong family history of migraine
b. frequently isolated to the occipital region
c. frequently associated with attention deficit hyperactivity disorder
d. duration of headache more than 24 h
e. rare termination by sleep

318. Examination of the cerebrospinal fluid of an 8-year-old, mildly febrile child with nuchal rigidity and intermittent stupor shows the following: white blood cells 100/mm^3 (all lymphocytes), negative Gram's stain, protein 150 mg/dL, and glucose 15 mg/dL. The most likely diagnosis is

a. tuberous sclerosis
b. tuberculous meningitis
c. stroke
d. acute bacterial meningitis
e. pseudotumor cerebri

319. A 6-year-old child has a somewhat unsteady but nonspecific gait and is irritable. Physical examination reveals a very mild left facial weakness, brisk stretch reflexes in all four extremities, bilateral extensor plantar responses (Babinski), and mild hypertonicity of the left upper and lower extremities; there is no muscular weakness. The most likely diagnosis is

a. pontine glioma
b. cerebellar astrocytoma
c. tumor of the right cerebral hemisphere
d. subacute sclerosing panencephalitis
e. subacute necrotizing leukoencephalopathy

320. A 2-year-old boy was just admitted to the hospital because of a convulsion 6 h ago followed by coma. The emergency room doctor ordered a CT scan with contrast, which showed enhancement of the basal cisterns by the contrast material. No other history is available. The most likely diagnosis is

a. battered child syndrome
b. malformation of the vein of Galen
c. meningococcal meningitis
d. tuberculous meningitis
e. eastern equine encephalitis

321. A 6-year-old child is hospitalized for observation because of a short period of unconsciousness after a fall from a playground swing. He has developed unilateral pupillary dilatation, focal seizures, recurrence of depressed consciousness, and hemiplegia. Appropriate management would be

a. spinal tap
b. CT scan
c. rapid fluid hydration
d. naloxone
e. gastric decontamination with charcoal

322. Headache, vomiting, and papilledema are common symptoms and signs in children who have brain tumors. Which of the following signs also is frequently associated with craniopharyngioma?

a. sixth-nerve palsy
b. unilateral cerebellar ataxia
c. unilateral pupillary dilatation
d. unilateral anosmia
e. bitemporal hemianopsia

323. A 6-year-old boy presents with the sudden onset of ataxia. Which of the following is the likely cause?

a. drug intoxication
b. agenesis of the corpus callosum
c. ataxia telangiectasia
d. muscular dystrophy
e. Friedreich's ataxia

324. Between 50 percent and 60 percent of tumors of the nervous system in children 2 to 12 years old are

a. subtentorial
b. supratentorial
c. intraventricular
d. in the spinal canal
e. none of the above

325. A young infant is noted to have facial diplegia and difficulty sucking and swallowing. The child has been colicky, and the maternal grandmother has been treating the child with a mixture of weak tea, rice water, and honey. Which of the following disorders is likely the culprit in this child?

a. infantile spinal muscular atrophy
b. myasthenia gravis
c. congenital myotonic dystrophy
d. Duchenne's muscular dystrophy
e. botulism

326. A cherry red spot in the eye is a well-known finding in Tay-Sachs disease. It may also be found in children with which of the following

a. Krabbe's disease
b. adrenoleukodystrophy
c. Rett syndrome
d. Gaucher's disease
e. metachromatic leukodystrophy

327. The true statement about simple febrile seizures includes which of the following?

a. there is usually a mild pleocytosis in the CSF
b. they usually occur in association with infections outside the central nervous system
c. they often last more than 15 min
d affected children usually are between 2 months and 10 years of age
e. focal activity is typical

328. The calcific densities in the skull x-ray shown below are likely to have been caused by

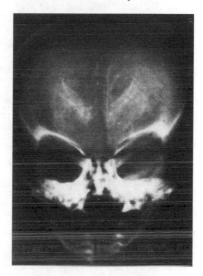

a. congenital cytomegalovirus infection
b. congenital toxoplasmosis
c. congenital syphilis
d. tuberculous meningitis
e. craniopharyngioma

329. The infant pictured develops infantile spasms. The disorder most likely to be affecting this infant is

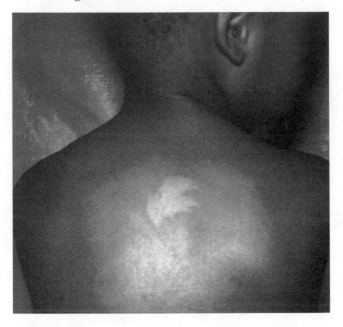

a. neurofibromatosis
b. tuberous sclerosis
c. incontinentia pigmenti
d. pityriasis rosea
e. psoriasis

330. A 4-year-old patient in coma with severe brain injury has developed diabetes insipidus with urine output of 100 mL/h. The diabetes insipidus can be managed by which of the following?

a. replacing excessive urine output with a solution of 5% glucose and normal saline
b. fluid restriction
c. oral (or nasogastric) hypoglycemic agents
d. giving insulin
e. giving DDAVP (synthetic vasopressin) intranasally

331. A 3-year-old boy's parents complain that their child has difficulty walking. The child rolled, sat, and first stood at essentially normal ages and first walked at 13 months of age. Over the past several months, the family has noticed an increased inward curvature of the lower spine as he walks and that his gait has become more "waddling" in nature. On examination, you confirm these later findings and also notice that he has enlargement of his calves. This child most likely has

a.   occult spina bifida
b.   muscular dystrophy
c.   brain tumor
d.   Guillain-Barré syndrome
e.   botulism

332. About 12 days after a mild upper respiratory infection, a 12-year-old boy complains of weakness in his lower extremities. Over several days, the weakness progresses to include his trunk. On physical examination, he has the weakness described and no lower extremity deep tendon reflexes, muscle atrophy, or pain. Spinal fluid studies are notable for elevated protein only. The most likely diagnosis in this patient is

a.   Bell's palsy
b.   muscular dystrophy
c.   Guillain-Barré syndrome
d.   Charcot-Marie-Tooth disease
e.   Werdnig-Hoffmann disease

Items 333–334

333. Your 6-year-old son awakens at 1:00 AM. screaming. You note that he is hyperventilating, is tachycardic, and has dilated pupils. He cannot be consoled, does not respond, and is unaware of his environment. After a few minutes, he returns to normal sleep. He recalls nothing the following morning. The most likely diagnosis is

a.   seizure disorder
b.   night terrors
c.   drug ingestion
d.   psychiatric disorder
e.   migraine headache

334. The most appropriate approach to this type of patient in the office setting is to

a.   obtain an EEG
b.   refer the patient to a child psychiatrist
c.   begin beta-blocker therapy
d.   reassure the patient and parents
e.   obtain a serum and urine drug screen

DIRECTIONS: Each group of questions below consists of lettered options followed by numbered items. For each numbered item, select the appropriate lettered option(s). Each lettered option may be used once, more than once, or not at all. **Choose exactly the number of options indicated following each item.**

Items 335–337

Certain arthropods elaborate venom that, when introduced into the human body, can be clinically important. For each arthropod, select the symptom or sign its venom is most likely to produce.

a. progressive paralysis
b. painful spasms of the abdominal muscles
c. chronic ulceration at the local site
d. only mild inflammation at the local site
e. a creeping eruption of the skin

335. Scorpion
(SELECT 1 FINDING)

336. Black widow spider
(SELECT 1 FINDING)

337. Tick **(SELECT 1 FINDING)**

Items 338–340

For each description, select the most likely diagnosis.

a. transient tic disorder of childhood
b. Tourette's syndrome
c. Sydenham's chorea
d. tardive dyskinesia
e. cerebral palsy

338. Eye blinking or throat clearing noises for a few months **(SELECT 1 DIAGNOSIS)**

339. May include motor and vocal tics **(SELECT 1 DIAGNOSIS)**

340. Nonprogressive disorder of movement and posture often found in association with visual, speech, and intellectual impairment **(SELECT 1 DIAGNOSIS)**

Items 341–343

For each diagnosis listed, select the most common clinical sign or symptom.

a. blindness of the affected side
b. ash leaf depigmentation
c. malignant neoplasm
d. increased incidence of infection
e. goiter

341. Neurofibromatosis type 1
(SELECT 1 FINDING)

342. McCune-Albright syndrome
(SELECT 1 FINDING)

343. Tuberous sclerosis
(SELECT 1 FINDING)

THE NEUROMUSCULAR SYSTEM

Answers

307. The answer is d. (*Behrman, 16/e, pp. 94–100. McMillan, 3/e, pp. 776–782. Rudolph, 20/e, pp. 121–128.*) Although early intervention is currently advocated for all of these conditions as soon as they are identified, studies of outcome are unable to validate that development is significantly improved in any but developmental language disorder. In support of such intervention is the fact that parental involvement is strengthened and parental needs supported. Developmental language disorder, if uncomplicated by other developmental impairments such as autism or mental retardation, is highly responsive to speech therapy, an intervention that can have long-term positive results.

308. The answer is d. (*Behrman, 16/e, p. 1961. McMillan, 3/e, p. 611. Rudolph, 20/e, pp. 1933–1934.*) The history, signs, and symptoms as outlined in the question are characteristic of a basilar skull fracture. Those patients with rupture of the tympanic membrane allowing otorrhea and those with rhinorrhea after the injury are at increased risk of complications of infection. For these children, a semi-upright position and observation for 72 h for evidence of increased intracranial pressure or infection without use of prophylactic antibiotics is appropriate. CSF drainage frequently stops within 72 h. Drainage beyond 72 h can require surgical closure; the risk of complications such as infection increases after this time.

309. The answer is e. (*Behrman, 16/e, pp. 1803–1806. McMillan, 3/e, pp. 223–224. Rudolph, 20/e, pp. 217, 1873.*) Mongolian spot is not related to any abnormality. Virtually any abnormality (except Mongolian spots) over the lower spine points to the possibility of occult spinal dysraphism. This designation includes a number of spinal cord and vertebral anomalies that frequently produce severe loss of neurologic function, particularly in the region of the back, the lower extremities, and the urinary system. Examples of these abnormalities are subcutaneous lipomeningomyelocele, diastematomyelia, hamartoma, lipoma, tight filum terminale, tethered cord, dermal and epidermal cysts, dermal sinuses, neurenteric canals, and angiomas. Occasionally, the loss of neurologic function from such anomalies is mild and as a result, easily overlooked. Prompt evaluation of these lesions via CT, MRI, or ultrasound is indicated.

310. The answer is b. *(Behrman, 16/e, pp. 344–347, 350–357, 373. McMillan, 3/e, pp. 1829–1830, 1832–1835, 1841–1842. Rudolph, 20/e, pp. 306–309, 311, 316–317, 320.)* Homocystinuria can cause thromboembolic phenomena in the pulmonary and systemic arteries and particularly in the cerebral vasculature; vascular occlusive disease is, in turn, one of the many causes of acute infantile hemiplegia. None of the other disorders listed in the question is associated with acute hemiplegia. Phenylketonuria causes retardation and, on occasion, seizures; maple syrup urine disease, an abnormality of the metabolism of leucine, leads to seizures and rapid deterioration of the central nervous system in newborn infants, histidinemia is associated with speech impairments and other minor neurologic difficulties; and cystathioninuria is most likely a benign aminoaciduria with no effect on the central nervous system.

311. The answer is e. *(Behrman, 16/e, pp. 1800–1801. McMillan, 3/e, pp. 2267–2268.)* In the infant, in contrast to the adult, it is often not possible to sense the sudden release of resistance that may occur as the needle penetrates the dura and enters the subarachnoid space. It is, therefore, very common for the physician not to realize that the tip of the needle is in the proper spot for fluid withdrawal and to mistakenly continue to advance the needle, which may penetrate a blood vessel, producing a traumatic tap and confusing the diagnosis. The stylet should be removed repeatedly as the needle is inserted to increase the chances that the fluid will be clear. Although not using a stylet at all can increase the chance of avoiding a traumatic tap, it produces the risk of inserting a core of epidermis into the subarachnoid space and producing an epidermoid tumor. The other wrong answers decrease the chances of success.

312. The answer is c. *(Behrman, 16/e, pp. 1885–1887. McMillan, 3/e, pp. 1967–1969. Rudolph, 20/e, pp. 1974–1976.)* Myasthenia gravis is usually an autoimmune disorder in which circulating acetylcholine receptor-binding antibodies are found in approximately 90 percent of cases, less commonly, when the patient demonstrates isolated eye disease. Other nonspecific evidence of autoimmune disease includes elevated ANAs, presence of abnormal immune complexes, and an association with the hypothyroidism related to lymphocytic thyroiditis, also an autoimmune disorder. The earliest signs of myasthenia gravis are ptosis and weakness of the extraocular muscles, followed by dysphagia and facial muscle weakness. The distinguishing hallmark of this disease is rapid fatiguing of the involved muscles. The conduction velocity of the motor nerve is normal in this condition. When the involved muscle is repetitively stimulated for diagnostic purposes, the EMG shows a decremental response, which can be reversed by the administration of cholinesterase inhibitors. These inhibitors are the primary therapeutic agents. Other therapeutic modalities for myasthenia gravis include immunosuppression, plasmapheresis, thymectomy (an enlarged thymus is frequently seen on chest x-ray), and treatment of hypothyroidism. CPK should be normal.

313. The answer is a. *(McMillan, 3/e, p. 1953.Rudolph, 20/e, pp. 2095–2096.)* Pinpoint pupils are found in coma, narcotics, pilocarpine, Horner's syndrome, pontine hemorrhage, posterior synechia formation, pesticide or nerve gas exposure, or in tertiary syphilis. Dilated pupils are seen with drugs such as epinephrine, phenylephrine, topical antihistamines/vasoconstrictor combinations and atropine-like agents. In addition, trauma, third nerve paralysis, or closed angle glaucoma can also cause pinpoint pupils

314. The answer is e.*(Behrman, 16/e, pp. 1854–1855. McMillan, 3/e, pp. 614–615, 1929, 1931–1933. Rudolph, 20/e, pp. 1877–1879, 1902–1903, 1924–1925, 1950, 1962–1963.)* The abrupt onset of a hemisyndrome, especially with the eyes looking away from the paralyzed side, strongly indicates a diagnosis of acute infantile hemiplegia. Most frequently, this represents a thromboembolic occlusion of the middle cerebral artery or one of its major branches. Hemiplegic migraine commonly occurs in children with a history of migraine headaches. Todd's paralysis follows after a focal or jacksonian seizure and generally does not last more than 24 to 48 h. The clinical onset of supratentorial brain tumor is subacute with repeated headaches and gradually developing weakness. A history of trauma usually precedes the signs of an acute subdural hematoma. Clinical signs of other diseases can appear fairly rapidly, but not often with the abruptness of occlusive vascular disease.

315. The answer is c. *(Behrman, 16/e, pp. 400, 1850. McMillan, 3/e, pp. 1875–1878. Rudolph, 20/e, pp. 335–336, 2025.)* Children who have Tay-Sachs disease are characterized by progressive developmental deterioration; physical signs include macular "cherry red" spots and exquisite sensitivity to noise. Diagnosis of this disorder can be confirmed biochemically by the absence of hexosaminidase A activity in white blood cells. Tay-Sachs disease is inherited as an autosomal recessive trait; frequently, affected children are of Eastern European Jewish ancestry. The other disorders listed in the question are associated with enzyme deficiencies as follows: Niemann-Pick disease, sphingomyelinase; infantile Gaucher's disease, beta-glucosidase; Krabbe's disease (globoid cell leukodystrophy), galactocerebroside beta-galactosidase; and Fabry's disease, alpha-galactosidase.

316. The answer is d. *(Behrman, 16/e, pp. 1878–1879. McMillan, 3/e, pp. 1973–1974. Rudolph, 20/e, pp. 1985–1986.)* Psychomotor retardation can be the presenting complaint of children who have myotonic dystrophy. Ptosis, baldness, hypogonadism, facial immobility with distal muscle wasting (in older children), and neonatal respiratory distress are major features of this disorder in the newborn period. Not infrequently, the mother will have the disease in a mild form, and a careful family history and examination of the parents, especially the mother, can be necessary to elicit the diagnosis, particularly since clinical and electrical evidence of myotonia may not be present in an affected infant. Seizures are not a feature of myotonic dystrophy.

317. The answer is a. *(Behrman, 16/e, pp. 1832–1834. McMillan, 3/e, pp. 679–680, 1931–1932, 2027–2029. Rudolph, 20/e, pp. 1962–1963.)* In contrast to adults, children with migraine most often have "common" migraine: bifrontal headache without an aura or diffuse throbbing headache of only a few hours' duration. As with adults, the headaches can be terminated with vomiting or sleep. Family history is frequently positive. Association with attention deficit hyperactivity disorder is not common, but a relationship with seizure disorder can be seen.

318. The answer is b. *(Behrman, 16/e p. 759. McMillan, 3/e, p. 859. Rudolph, 20/e, pp. 618, 636, 1920–1922.)* Included among those things that can cause the clinical picture are viral meningitis, tuberculous meningitis, meningeal leukemia, and medulloblastoma, all of which can cause pleocytosis as well as elevated protein and lowered glucose concentrations in cerebrospinal fluid. Of the four diseases (and the likely finding of this patient), tuberculous meningitis is associated with the lowest glucose levels in cerebrospinal fluid. The cellular response to viral meningitis eventually will be predominantly lymphocytic. Cells found in the cerebrospinal fluid of a child who has meningeal leukemia most commonly are lymphocytes or lymphoblasts. Children who have a medulloblastoma generally present with the signs and symptoms caused by a mass in the posterior cranial fossa; their pleocytotic cerebrospinal fluid contains unusual-appearing cells of the monocytic variety. The decrease in the glucose concentration of cerebrospinal fluid associated with these disorders has been attributed to a disturbance of glucose transport as a result of meningeal irritation. In pseudotumor cerebri, the constituents of cerebrospinal fluid are generally normal except for a low protein content in some instances. Acute bacterial disease typically causes polymorphonuclear cells and positive Gram's stains. Neither tuberous sclerosis nor stroke typically cause these findings on CFS examination.

319. The answer is a. *(Behrman, 16/e pp. 1858–1862. McMillan, 3/e, pp. 1511–1515. Rudolph, 20/e, pp. 1900–1913.)* A child who has a subacute disorder of the central nervous system that produces cranial nerve abnormalities (especially of cranial nerve VII and the lower bulbar nerves), long-tract signs, unsteady gait secondary to spasticity, and some behavioral changes is most likely to have a pontine glioma. Tumors of the cerebellar hemispheres can, in later stages, produce upper motor neuron signs, but the gait disturbance would be ataxia. Dysmetria and nystagmus also would be present. Supratentorial tumors are quite uncommon in 6-year-old children; headache and vomiting would be likely presenting symptoms and papilledema a finding on physical examination.

320. The answer is d. *(Behrman, 16/e pp. 890–891. McMillan, 3/e, p. 1033. Rudolph, 20/e, p. 618.)* The CT scan with contrast can be an excellent clue for diagnosing tuberculous meningitis. Exudate in the basal cisterns that shows enhancement by contrast material is typical; tuberculomas, lucencies, edema, and infarction can be apparent; and hydrocephalus can develop. Confirmation with culture is mandatory. The x-ray of the chest will be likely to show signs of pulmonary tuberculosis. A high index of suspicion is necessary to diagnose tuberculous meningitis early.

321. The answer is b. *(Behrman, 16/e pp. 272–273. McMillan, 3/e, pp. 614–615. Rudolph, 20/e, p. 1937.)* Compression of cranial nerve III and distortion of the brainstem, resulting in unilateral pupillary dilatation, hemiplegia, focal seizures, and depressed consciousness, suggest a progressively enlarging mass, most likely a subdural hematoma. Such a hematoma displaces the temporal lobe into the tentorial notch and presses on the ipsilateral cranial nerve III. Brainstem compression by this additional tissue mass leads to progressive deterioration in consciousness. Rising blood pressure and falling pulse rate are characteristic of increasing intracranial pressure. The most urgent test to diagnose this condition is a CT scan.

322. The answer is e. *(Behrman, 16/e, p. 1861. Rudolph, 20/e, pp. 1915–1916.)* Upward growth of a craniopharyngioma results in compression of the optic chiasm. Particularly affected are the fibers derived from the nasal portions of both retinas (in other words, from those parts of the eyes receiving stimulation from the temporal visual field). Early in the growth of a craniopharyngioma, a unilateral superior quadrantanopsic defect can develop; and an irregularly growing tumor can impinge upon the optic chiasm and cause homonymous hemianopia.

323. The answer is a. *(Behrman, 16/e pp. 1839–1840. Rudolph, 20/e, pp. 1866, 2057–2058.)* Cerebellar ataxia in childhood can occur in association with infection, metabolic abnormalities, ingestion of toxins, hydrocephalus, cerebellar lesions, multiple sclerosis, labyrinthitis, polyradiculopathy, and neuroblastoma. Although the other diagnoses (except agenesis of the corpus collasum) can cause ataxia, it is more of a chronic nature than acute. Ingestion (intentional or accidental) of barbiturates, phenytoin, alcohol, and other drugs also must be considered. Agenesis of the corpus callosum is usually diagnosed by imaging studies; however, it does not cause acute ataxia.

324. The answer is a. *(Behrman, 16/e pp. 1858–1862. McMillan, 3/e, pp. 1511–1513. Rudolph, 20/e, pp. 1900–1905.)* Approximately two thirds of intracranial tumors in children are located below the tentorium. Of these tumors, the two most common types are medulloblastoma and cerebellar astrocytoma. In adults and infants, most intracranial tumors originate above the tentorium; only 25 percent to 30 percent of brain tumors in adults are subtentorial.

325. The answer is e. *(Behrman, 16/e pp. 875–878. McMillan, 3/e, p. 941. Rudolph, 20/e, pp. 1968–1970.)* Spinal muscular atrophy in a neonate is associated with hypotonia and feeding difficulties; a muscle biopsy can confirm this diagnosis. Neonatal myasthenia gravis and botulism, though uncommon, must be considered in a newborn infant who has the symptoms described in the question. The symptoms presented also could represent myotonic dystrophy; this diagnosis is confirmed by examination of both parents for percussion and grip myotonia and by electromyographic depiction of myotonic discharges. Duchenne's (pseudohypertrophic) muscular dystrophy clinically appears in children who are about 2 or 3 years of age. Botulism has clearly been associated with the ingestion of raw honey. In this child, while the other possibilities listed in the question may be the etiology, it seems most likely that botulism is the culprit.

326. The answer is d. *(Behrman, 16/e p. 1928. McMillan, 3/e, pp. 1875–1878, 1993–1995, 2004–2005. Rudolph, 20/e, pp. 334–341, 1898–1899.)* The cherry red spot represents the center of a normal retinal macula that is surrounded by ganglion cells in which there is an abnormal accumulation of lipid. This alters the surrounding retinal color so that it is yellowish or grayish white. It can be seen in such disorders as GM_1 generalized gangliosidosis type 1, Sandhoff disease, and Niemann Pick disease type A, in which there is lipid material deposited in the ganglion cells. Metachromatic leukodystrophy does not affect the retina as it is a demyelinating disorder rather than a "storage" disease.

327. The answer is b. *(Behrman, 16/e, pp. 1818–1819. McMillan, 3/e, pp. 1949–1952 Rudolph, 20/e, pp. 1965–1966.)* Febrile seizures usually occur in children between the ages of 9 months and 5 years and generally in association with upper respiratory illness, roseola, shigellosis, or gastroenteritis. The generalized seizures are mostly brief (2 to 5 min) and the cerebrospinal fluid is normal. Infants who have seizures that are prolonged (longer than 15 min), focal, or lateralized, or who had neurologic problems before the febrile seizure, are at a higher risk of developing an afebrile seizure disorder during the next 5 to 7 years.

328. The answer is a. *(Behrman, 16/e, pp. 981–984, 1054–1062. McMillan, 3/e, pp. 429–433, 445–447, 1033. Rudolph, 20/e, pp. 629–633, 768–772.)* Periventricular calcifications are a characteristic finding in infants who have congenital cytomegalovirus infection. The encephalitic process especially affects the subependymal tissue around the lateral ventricles and thus, results in the periventricular deposition of calcium. Calcified tuberculomas, if visible radiographically, are not particularly periventricular. Granulomatous encephalitis caused by congenital toxoplasmosis is associated with scattered and soft-appearing intracranial calcification, and suprasellar calcifications are typical of craniopharyngiomas. Congenital syphilis does not produce intracranial calcifications.

329. The answer is b. *(Behrman, 16/e, p. 1837. McMillan, 3/e, pp. 2023–2024. Rudolph, 20/e, pp. 2043–2044.)* In infants, achromic skin patches, especially in association with infantile spasms, are characteristic of tuberous sclerosis. Other dermal abnormalities (adenoma sebaceum and subungual fibromata) associated with this disorder appear later in childhood. Although children who have neurofibromatosis may have a few achromic patches, the identifying dermal lesions are café au lait spots. Incontinentia pigmenti also is associated with seizures; the skin lesions typical of this disorder begin as bullous eruptions that later become hyperpigmented lesions. Pityriasis rosea and psoriasis are not associated with infantile spasms.

330. The answer is e. *(Behrman, 16/e, pp. 195–196, 1681–1683. McMillan, 3/e, pp. 1783, 1792, 1955. Rudolph, 20/e, pp. 1705–1708.)* Diabetes insipidus is a common complication of severe head trauma and is due to a deficiency in secretion of antidiuretic hormone. It must be distinguished from the polyuria that can occur several days after head injury, as the high antidiuretic hormone levels associated with the head injury, resolve. This form of diabetes insipidus can be treated by replacement of urinary losses intravenously or enterally with solutions low in sodium as long as it is possible to keep up with the losses. Vasopressin given intramuscularly or as an intranasal preparation makes care easier and safer as long as water balance is carefully monitored.

331. The answer is b. *(Behrman, 16/e, pp. 1873–1877. McMillan, 3/e, pp. 1972–1976. Rudolph, 20/e, pp. 1979–1981.)* The most common form of muscular dystrophy is Duchenne's muscular dystrophy. It is inherited as an X-linked recessive trait. Male infants are rarely diagnosed at birth or early infancy since they often reach gross milestones at the expected age.

Early after walking, however, the features of this disease become more evident. While these children walk at the appropriate age, the hip girdle weakness is seen by age 2. Increased lordosis when standing is evidence of gluteal weakness. Gowers' sign (use of the hands to "climb up" the legs in order to assume the upright position) is seen by 3 to 5 years of age as is the hip waddle gait. Ambulation ability remains through about 7 to 12 years, after which use of a wheelchair is common. Associated features include mental impairment and cardiomyopathy. Death due to respiratory failure, heart failure, pneumonia, or aspiration is common by 18 years of age.

332. The answer is c. *(Behrman, 16/e, pp. 1892–1893. McMillan, 3/e, pp. 1962–1963. Rudolph, 20/e, pp. 1668, 1970–1972.)* The paralysis of Guillain-Barré occurs about 10 days after a nonspecific viral illness. Weakness is gradual over days or weeks beginning in the lower extremities and progresses toward the trunk. Later, the upper limbs and the bulbar muscles can become involved. Involvement of the respiratory muscles is life-threatening. The syndrome seems to be caused by a demyelination in the motor and occasionally, the sensory, nerves. Spinal fluid protein is helpful in the diagnosis; protein levels are increased to more than twice normal, while glucose and cell counts are normal. Hospitalization for observation is indicated. Treatment can consist of intravenous immunoglobulin, steroids, or plasmapheresis. Recovery is not always complete.

333–334. The answers are 333–b, 334–d. *(Behrman, 16/e, pp. 16, 1829. McMillan, 3/e, p. 826. Rudolph, 20/e, pp. 25, 101–102, 1960.)* Night terrors are most common in boys between the ages of 5 and 7 years. The child awakens suddenly, appears frightened and unaware of his surroundings, and has the clinical signs outlined in the question. He cannot be consoled by the parents. After a few minutes, sleep follows and the patient cannot recall the event in the morning. Sleepwalking is common in these children. Exploring the family dynamics for emotional disorders may be helpful; usually pharmacologic therapy is not required and family reassurance is indicated.

335–337. The answers are 335–a, 336–b, 337–a. *(Behrman, 16/e, pp. 1887, 2175–2177. McMillan, 3/e, pp. 1209–1210, 1970–1971. Rudolph, 20/e, pp. 779–782.)* Both scorpions and ticks can produce progressive ascending paralysis. The tick paralysis is trickier to diagnose because the only sign of illness can be the paralysis. It can be caused by such ticks as the eastern dog or the Rocky Mountain wood tick, which inject toxin in their saliva while they remain attached. They should be aggressively sought since removal usually brings cure and averts possible death. The scorpion sting is usually easier to diagnose since scorpions are easier to see and the sting induces a severe reaction with pain and swelling and can also induce a severe systemic reaction with shock, excessive salivation, and convulsions. In addition to supportive therapy, including the use of tourniquets and phenobarbital (but not morphine), specific antivenins are available.

Black widow spiders are also capable of making their presence known not only by their distinctive markings, but also by their ability to attract one's attention to the site of their bite by a marked, painful local reaction followed by a systemic reaction with nausea, vomiting, sweating, hypertension, and cramping abdominal pain. Pain can be treated with meperidine (Demerol) or intravenous calcium gluconate, and a specific antivenin should be used.

338–340. The answers are 338–a, 339–b, 340–e. *(Behrman, 16/e, pp. 1842–1845. McMillan, 3/e, pp. 1910–1917, 2014–2015. Rudolph, 20/e, pp. 1892–1896, 1960, 2040.)* Tics are commonly seen in a pediatric practice. All have in common the nonrhythmic, spasmodic, involuntary, stereotypical behaviors that involve any muscle group. Transient tic disorder is the most common and is seen more often in boys; a family history is often noted. In this condition, the patient has eye-blinking, facial movements, or throat clearing lasting for weeks to about a year. No medications are needed. Chronic motor tics persist throughout life and can involve motor movements involving up to three muscle groups.

Gilles de la Tourette's syndrome is a life-long condition that is characterized by motor and vocal tics, obsessive-compulsive behavior, and a high incidence of attention-deficit disorder with hyperactivity (ADDH). Therapy for the ADDH is helpful, as is medication to control the motor or vocal tics. Multiple psychosocial problems exist with these children; a multidisciplinary approach is helpful.

Cerebral palsy is a static condition of movement and posture disorders frequently associated with epilepsy and abnormalities of vision, speech, and intellect. A defect in the developing brain is felt to be the cause. No significant change in the incidence of cerebral palsy has been noted in the past few decades despite drastically improved obstetric and neonatal care. No treatment of cerebral palsy is available; a multidisciplinary approach to manage the many medical problems associated with the condition is helpful.

341–343. The answers are 341–c, 342–e, 343–b. (*Behrman, 16/e, pp. 1692–1693, 1835–1837. McMillan, 3/e, p. 2026. Rudolph, 20/e, pp. 429–430, 904–905, 2043–2048.*) Tuberous sclerosis, an autosomal dominant condition, can result in severe mental retardation and seizures. Infantile spasms, a hypsarrhythmic EEG pattern, hypopigmented lesions (ash leaf spots), cardiac tumors, sebaceous adenomas, a shagreen patch (a roughened, raised lesion over the sacrum), and calcifications on the CT scan are all features of this condition. No specific treatment is available.

Neurofibromatosis type 1 (NF1) is a progressive neurocutaneous syndrome that results from a defect in neural crest differentiation and migration during the early stages of development. It has an autosomal dominant pattern of inheritance; the gene locus has been identified on chromosome 17. Any organ or system can be affected, neurologic complications are frequent, and patients are at high risk of developing malignant neoplasms of various types. The presence of any two of the following findings confirms the diagnosis of NF1.

1.   Five or more café au lait spots over 5 mm in diameter in prepubertal patients; six or more over 15 mm in diameter in postpubertal patients
2.   Axillary freckling
3.   Two or more Lisch nodules (hamartomas of the iris)
4.   Two or more neurofibromas, typically involving the skin and appearing during adolescence or pregnancy; or one plexiform neuroma involving a nerve track present at birth
5.   Bony lesions leading to pathologic fracture and kyphoscoliosis
6.   Optic glioma
7.   NF1 in a first-degree relative

McCune-Albright syndrome and NF1 share many of the same clinical findings: skin, bones, and endocrine glands can be involved in both. The characteristic features of McCune-Albright syndrome include large, irregular, usually unilateral café au lait spots and fibrous dysplasia of bones in association with precocious puberty in girls. Although the last finding has been the major recognized endocrinopathy in the syndrome, disorders of pituitary, thyroid, and adrenal have been noted with greater frequency in recent years. The endocrinopathies are ascribed to autonomous hyperfunctioning of the involved gland with goiter.

INFECTIOUS DISEASES AND IMMUNOLOGY

Questions

DIRECTIONS: Each item below contains a question or incomplete statement followed by suggested responses. Select the **one best** response to each question.

344. Which of the following infections typically has an incubation period of less than 2 weeks?

a. mumps
b. varicella
c. rubella
d. measles
e. rabies

345. The care of children with AIDS includes which of the following?

a. monthly evaluation for Kaposi's sarcoma
b. prophylaxis against *Pneumocystis carinii* pneumonia (PCP)
c. vitamin C supplementation
d. oral polio virus
e. bone marrow transplantation

346. Influenza virus vaccine is usually administered annually because of antigen shift and limited duration of protection. Which of the groups below should receive the vaccine?

a. infant with Still's murmur
b. government employees
c. infants under 6 months of age
d. patients on long-term aspirin therapy
e. young patients with seizure disorder

347. An 18-month-old child presents to the emergency center having had a brief, generalized tonic-clonic seizure. He is now postictal and has a temperature of 40°C (104°F). During the lumbar puncture (which proves to be normal), he has a large, watery stool that has both blood and mucus in it. The most likely diagnosis in this patient is

a. *Salmonella*
b. enterovirus
c. rotavirus
d. *Campylobacter*
e. *Shigella*

348. Scarlet fever and Kawasaki syndrome have many manifestations in common. Which of the following statements comparing these diseases is true?

a. neither has cardiac complications
b. serologic tests are helpful in diagnosing both
c. Kawasaki syndrome has mucocutaneous and lymph node involvement but scarlet fever does not
d. pharyngeal culture aids in the diagnosis of scarlet fever but not Kawasaki syndrome
e. a specific therapy is recommended for scarlet fever but supportive care only is recommended for Kawasaki syndrome

349. A patient with hair loss is shown below. The lesion does not fluoresce with a Wood's lamp and has not responded well to a variety of topical agents. The lesion is boggy, is spreading, and has tiny pinpoint black dots throughout the lesion. The most likely diagnosis is

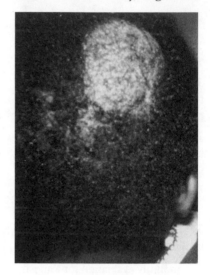

a. traction alopecia
b. infection with *Trichophyton tonsurans*
c. alopecia areata
d. biotinidase deficiency
e. hypothyroidism

350. Which of the following viruses has been implicated in causing erythema infectiosum, transient aplastic anemia, persistent infection in patients with immunodeficiency, and hydrops fetalis?

a. roseola
b. parvovirus B-19
c. Coxsackie A-16
d. Echovirus 11
e. Cytomegalovirus

Items 351–352

351. A 17-year-old male complains of acute, painful, scrotal swelling. Ultrasound of the testes is normal, but the urinalysis reveals pyuria. The most likely diagnosis in this patient is

a. incarcerated inguinal hernia
b. torsion of the testes
c. varicocele
d. epididymitis
e. urinary tract infection

352. Appropriate therapy for this patient is

a. surgical consultation
b. culture, intramuscular ceftriaxone, and oral doxycycline
c. voiding cystourethrogram
d. oral sulfonamides for 3 days
e. warm compresses and counseling

353. A 15-month-old boy is brought to the emergency room because of fever and a rash. Six hours earlier he was fine, except for tugging on his ears; another physician diagnosed otitis media and prescribed amoxicillin. During the interim period, the child has developed an erythematous rash on his face, trunk, and extremities. Some of the lesions, which are of variable size, do not blanch on pressure. The child is now very irritable and he does not interact well with the examiner. Temperature is 39.5°C (103.1°F). He continues to have injected, immobile tympanic membranes. The most appropriate next step in the management of this infant is to

a. begin administration of intravenous ampicillin
b. begin diphenhydramine
c. discontinue administration of ampicillin and begin trimethoprim with sulfamethoxazole
d. perform bilateral myringotomies
e. perform a lumbar picture

354. The 3-year-old sister of a newborn baby develops a cough diagnosed as pertussis by nasopharyngeal culture. The mother gives a history of having been immunized as a child. A correct statement regarding this clinical situation is

a.   the mother has no risk of acquiring the disease because she was immunized

b.   hyperimmune globulin is effective in protecting the infant

c.   the risk to the infant depends on the immune status of the mother

d.   erythromycin should be administered to the infant

e.   the 3-year-old sister should be immediately immunized with an additional dose of pertussis vaccine

355. A 14-year-old boy is seen in the emergency room because of a 3-week history of fever between 38.3°C and 38.9°C (101°F and 102°F), lethargy, and a 6-lb weight loss. Physical examination reveals marked cervical and inguinal adenopathy, enlarged tonsils with exudate, small hemorrhages on the soft palate, a WBC differential that has 50 percent lymphocytes (10 percent atypical), and a palpable spleen 2 cm below the left costal margin. Which of the following conditions is the likely diagnosis?

a.   HIV disease
b.   varicella
c.   Kawasaki disease
d.   streptococcal throat infection
e.   infectious mononucleosis

356. Which of the following statements about acute osteomyelitis is correct?

a.   it most commonly is caused by *Streptococcus pyogenes*

b.   it often arises following development of deep cellulitis

c.   tenderness in the region of infection is diffuse, not localized

d.   bony changes are visible radiographically within 48 hours of the beginning of symptoms

e.   antibiotic therapy usually is required for at 10 to 14 days

357. A 16-day-old infant presents with fever, irritability, poor feeding, and a bulging fontanelle. Spinal fluid demonstrates gram-positive cocci. The most likely diagnosis is ·

a.   *Listeria monocytogenes*
b.   group A streptococcus
c.   group B streptococcus
d.   *Streptococcus pneumoniae*
e.   *Staphylococcus aureus*

358. Which of the following statements regarding infant botulism is correct?

a.   findings on physical examination include diffuse hypertonia and increased deep tendon reflexes

b.   most surviving infants have residual neurologic damage

c.   the spores of *Clostridium botulinum* germinate in the infant's intestine

d.   the spores have been found in rice water

e.   it is a distinct syndrome consisting of diarrhea, hyperphagia, tachycardia, and irritability

359. A 14-month-old infant suddenly develops a fever of 40.2°C (104.4°F). Physical examination shows an alert, active infant who drinks milk eagerly. No physical abnormalities are noted. The white blood cell count is 22,000/mm^3 with 78 percent polymorphonuclear leukocytes, 18 percent of which are band forms. The most likely diagnosis is

a. pneumococcal bacteremia
b. roseola
c. streptococcosis
d. typhoid fever
e. diphtheria

360. When the mother contracts German measles (rubella) early in pregnancy, effects on the fetus may commonly include which of the following?

a. thrombocytosis
b. wide-set eyes
c. glaucoma
d. tetrology of Fallot
e. duodenal atresia

361. The 3-year-old boy seen in the following photograph is brought to the emergency room with a swollen eye. He was well until 3 days ago when he developed symptoms of an upper respiratory infection, which gradually worsened. On the night before admission, he was noted to have a temperature of 39.6°C (103.3°F). The child presents with proptosis, limitation of eye movement, chemosis, and decreased visual acuity. Your diagnosis for this patient is

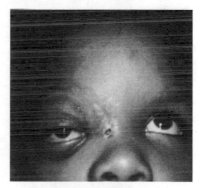

(Courtesy Binita Shah, M.D.)

a. retinoblastoma
b. periorbital cellulitis
c. glaucoma
d. orbital cellulitis
e. myasthenia gravis

362. The pictured child presents with a 3-day history of malaise, fever to 106°F, cough, coryza, and conjunctivitis. He then develops the erythematous, maculopapular rash pictured. He is noted to have white pinpoint lesions on a bright red buccal mucosa in the area opposite his lower molars. The most likely diagnosis is

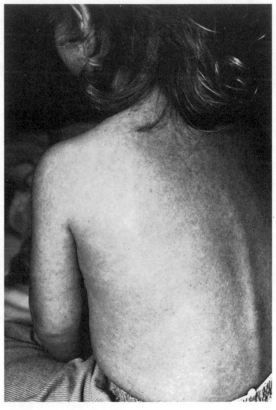

(Courtesy Adelaide Hebert, M.D.)

a.   parvovirus
b.   rubella
c.   herpes
d.   roseola
e.   varicella

363. A 3-year-old child awakens at night with a fever of 39.6°C (103.3°F), a severe sore throat, and a barking cough. Physical examination of the child, who is drooling, shows a very red throat and inspiratory stridor. Optimal management would include

a.   immediate hospitalization for possible intubation
b.   immediate inhalation therapy with racemic epinephrine
c.   treatment with oral ampicillin, 50 mg/kg per day
d.   suctioning of the pharynx and hourly examinations of the hypopharynx
e.   a throat culture and expectorant and mist therapy

364. A 14-year-old girl awakens with a mild sore throat, low-grade fever, and a diffuse maculopapular rash. During the next 24 h, she develops tender swelling of her wrists and redness of her eyes. In addition, her physician notes mild tenderness and marked swelling of her posterior cervical and occipital lymph nodes. Four days after the onset of her illness, the rash has vanished. The most likely diagnosis of this girl's condition is

a.   rubella
b.   rubeola
c.   roseola
d.   erythema infectiosum
e.   erythema multiforme

365. A 4-year-old child presents in the clinic with mumps. Correct statements about this condition include which of the following?

a.   arthritis is a common presenting complaint in children
b.   the disease could have been prevented by prior immunization with killed whole cell vaccine
c.   involvement of the CNS may occur 10 days after the resolution of the parotitis
d.   orchitis occurs almost exclusively in prepubertal males
e.   subendocardial fibroelastosis is a common complication in this age child

366. Common features of infection with hepatitis A virus include which of the following?

a.   long incubation period (50 to 80 days)
b.   prolonged viremia
c.   presentation with the sudden onset of fever, nausea, and vomiting
d.   transmission by parenteral route
e.   prolonged elevations of SGOT and serum bilirubin for 6 months or more

367. Which of the following is a contraindication to lumbar puncture in a 9-month-old infant with suspected meningitis?

a.   uncorrected bleeding diathesis
b.   bulging fontanelle
c.   lumbar puncture 2 days before
d.   marked uncooperativeness on the part of the patient
e.   significantly elevated WBC count consistent with bacteremia

368. A 6-year-old comes to the clinic with the rapid onset of fever, muscle pain, and rash. The rash that developed is maculopapular, beginning on the flexor surfaces of the wrist and evolving to a hemor-rhagic-type appearance. The history is positive for his going camping with the Boy Scouts 9 days prior to presentation. Ticks were found on several of the campers. Which of the following is likely?

a.   Lyme disease
b.   tularemia
c.   measles
d.   toxic shock syndrome
e.   Rocky Mountain spotted fever

369. Concerning a positive Mantoux (PPD) test in a child, which of the following statements is true?

a.   it generally develops within 2 to 5 days after infection
b.   it indicates that the child is contagious
c.   it rarely indicates a need for antimicrobial therapy
d.   it usually reverts to negative after 6 months
e.   it may indicate infection with atypical mycobacteria

370. The rash and mucous membrane lesions shown in the photograph develop in an infant 5 days after a nonspecific upper respiratory tract infection. Which of the following is LEAST likely to be responsible?

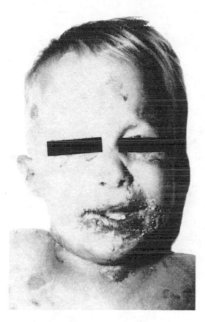

a. *Mycoplasma pneumoniae*
b. Herpesvirus hominis type 1
c. Rubella virus
d. phenytoin ingestion
e. penicillin therapy

371. Which of the following parasites typically produce disease in the course of their migration through the parenchyma of body tissues?

a. *Cryptosporidium parvum*
b. *Sporothrix schenckii*
c. *Giardia lambila*
d. *Enterobius vermicularis*
e. *Trichinella spiralis*

372. A 10-year-old boy from the Connecticut coast is seen because of discomfort in his right knee. He had a large, annular, erythematous lesion on his back that disappeared 4 weeks prior to the present visit. His mother recalls pulling a small tick off his back. The correct statement about this child's likely illness includes which of the following?

a. The tick was probably a *Dermacentur andersoni*
b. The disease is caused by a rickettsial agent that is transmitted by the bite of a tick
c. In addition to skin and joint involvement, CNS and cardiac abnormalities may be present
d. Therapy with antibiotics has little effect on the resolution of symptoms
e. The pathognomonic skin lesion is required for diagnosis

373. The 6-year-old patient pictured presents with a 6 h history of fever to 102°F. Her mother reports that the patient was complaining of not feeling well, that she had a headache, and she was nauseated. About 2 hours prior to arrival to the emergency room, the mother states that she noted a few purple spots scattered about the body on the patient, especially on the buttocks and legs. On the 30 min ride to the emergency room, the rash has spread rapidly as shown and the patient is now obtunded. Of the following, the most likely diagnosis is

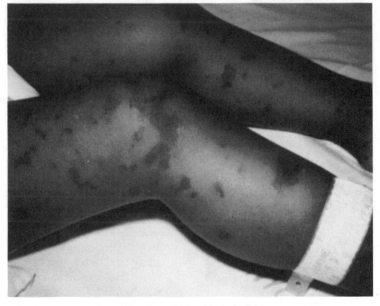

(Courtesy Binita Shah, M.D.)

a. Stevens-Johnson syndrome
b. toxic shock syndrome caused by *Staphylococcus aureus*
c. measles
d. Rocky Mountain spotted fever
e. meningococcemia

374. A child with viral croup can be expected to have which of the following?

a. a temperature greater than 102°F
b. expiratory stridor
c. infection with parainfluenza virus
d. hyperinflation on chest x-ray
e. age between 6 years and 8 years

375. Two weeks ago, a 5-year-old boy developed diarrhea, which has persisted to the present time, despite dietary management. His stools have been watery, pale, and frothy. He has been afebrile. Microscopic examination of his stools is likely to show which of the following?

a. *Salmonella sonnei*
b. *Enterobius vermicularis*
c. *Sporothrix schencki*
d. *Toxoplasma gondii*
e. *Cryptosporidium*

DIRECTIONS: Each group of questions below consists of lettered options followed by numbered items. For each numbered item, select the appropriate lettered option(s). Each lettered option may be used once, more than once, or not at all. **Choose exactly the number of options indicated following each item.**

Items 376–379

For each set of immunologic abnormalities listed in the table below, **SELECT 1 DIAGNOSIS.**

a. Bruton disease
b. DiGeorge anomaly
c. Wiskott-Aldrich syndrome
d. Job-Buckley syndrome
e. Swiss-type immunodeficiency disease (severe combined immunodeficiency disease [SCID])

	Serum IgG	Serum IgA	Serum IgM	T-Cell Function	Parathyroid Function
376.	Normal	Normal	Normal	Decreased	Decreased
377.	Low	Low	Low	Normal	Normal
378.	Low	Low	Low	Decreased	Normal
379.	Normal	High	Low	Decreased	Normal

Items 380–385

Match the disease with the associated organism.

a. *Rochalimaea henselae*
b. *Pseudomonas*
c. Rubivirus
d. human herpesvirus 6
e. *Escherichia coli*
f. *Helicobacter pylori*

g. group B streptococci
h. *Listeria monocytogenes*
i. Epstein-Barr virus
j. *Toxocara cati*
k. *Campylobacter jejuni*

380. Cystic fibrosis **(SELECT 1 ORGANISM)**

381. Foot puncture wound through tennis shoe **(SELECT 1 ORGANISM)**

382. Cat-scratch disease **(SELECT 1 ORGANISM)**

383. Roseola **(SELECT 1 ORGANISM)**

384. Burns **(SELECT 1 ORGANISM)**

385. Peptic ulcer **(SELECT 1 ORGANISM)**

Items 386–388

Match the diagnostic test with the associated disease state.

a. herpes simplex
b. fungal infection
c. bacterial infection
d. worm infestation
e. malarial infection

386. Wood's lamp
(SELECT 1 DISEASE)

387. Tzanck's smear
(SELECT 1 DISEASE)

388. Scotch tape preparation
(SELECT 1 DISEASE)

Items 389–392

Match each clinical state with the most likely form of pneumonia.

a. mycoplasmal pneumonia
b. pneumococcal pneumonia
c. chlamydial pneumonia
d. viral pneumonia
e. tuberculous pneumonia
f. fungal pneumonia
g. staphylococcal pneumonia

389. A 6-week-old infant with tachypnea and history of eye discharge at 2 weeks of age
(SELECT 1 DIAGNOSIS)

390. A 14-year-old girl with low-grade fever, cough of 3 weeks' duration, and interstitial pneumonia
(SELECT 1 DIAGNOSIS)

391. A 2-month-old boy with a 3-day history of upper respiratory infection who suddenly develops high fever, cough, and respiratory distress; within 48 h, the patient has developed a pneumatocele and a left-sided pneumothorax
(SELECT 1 DIAGNOSIS)

392. An 8-year-old girl with fever, tachypnea, and interstitial infiltrate and hilar adenopathy on chest x-ray; her social history is positive for an uncle living in the home who has a cough and recently released from prison
(SELECT 1 DIAGNOSIS)

INFECTIOUS DISEASES AND IMMUNOLOGY

Answers

344. The answer is d. *(Behrman, 16/e, pp. 946–955, 973–977, 1014–1017. McMillan 3/e, pp. 1127–1130, 1134–1142. Rudolph, 20/e, pp. 661–671, 679–681, 684–686.)* The usual incubation periods of several important diseases are as follows: measles, 10 to 12 days; varicella, 11 to 20 days; rubella, 14 to 21 days; mumps, 12 to 22 days; and rabies, 9 days to several months or years (average 18 to 60 days). The durations of infectivity are as follows: measles, from 2 days before the onset of the catarrhal stage through the third through fifth day of the rash; varicella, from 2 days before the eruption until the last vesicle has dried (approximately 5 to 7 days); rubella, from 7 days before the onset of the rash to up to 7 to 8 days after its onset (infants with congenital rubella may excrete the virus for more than 1 year); mumps, from 2 days before until 9 days after the onset of parotid swelling.

345. The answer is b. *(Behrman, 16/e, pp. 1022–1032. McMillan 3/e, pp. 867–893. Rudolph, 20/e, pp. 655–660.)* The severe anemia associated with AIDS can require blood transfusion, especially if there is evidence of respiratory compromise. Donor blood should be CMV-negative to avoid CMV infection, a serious and possibly fatal disease in the immunocompromised patient.

AIDS patients should receive primary and booster immunization with diphtheria-pertussis-tetanus (DPT), MMR, hepatitis B, and *Haemophilus influenzae* type B conjugated vaccine (HibCV). Inactivated polio vaccine (IPV) is recommended in place of oral polio vaccine (OPV) because of the theoretical risk of paralytic polio. Although vaccination with MMR is precluded in other immunodeficient patients, those with AIDS should be immunized against measles, mumps, and rubella. The morbidity and mortality associated with these diseases in AIDS patients significantly override the risk of vaccine complications. If these children are exposed to measles, they should receive a protective dose of measles immunoglobulin regardless of their immunization history. Pneumovax at age 2 and influenza vaccine are recommended annually .

The drug of choice for treatment of *Pneumocystis carinii* pneumonia (PCP) is trimethoprim-sulfamethoxazole. In certain situations, it is used as prophylaxis against PCP infection in patients with AIDS.

Eventually, all patients infected with HIV will lose weight and fail to grow. The factors responsible include reduced caloric intake because of poor appetite, intestinal malabsorption, and increased resting energy expenditure associated with chronic infection. Maintaining adequate nutrition in AIDS patients is very difficult. Vitamin C supplementation, by itself, has no special benefits.

Bone marrow transplants in AIDS patients have been unsuccessful thus far because of the persistence of virus in macrophages throughout the body. Kaposi's sarcoma is rare in children.

346. The answer is d. *(Behrman, 16/e, p. 989. McMillan 3/e, pp. 1083, 1089–1091. Rudolph, 20/e, pp. 676–677.)* Patients targeted to receive this vaccine are those with chronic cardiac, pulmonary, hematologic, and neurologic problems in which respiratory compromise is part of the syndrome, as well as children with symptomatic HIV infection. Sound immunization practice regarding influenza stresses the importance of immunizing not only the high-risk patient but also all close contacts and medical personnel. Health professionals are at increased risk of exposure to influenza, and in the event of an epidemic, their absence from work because of illness would seriously compromise patient care. Reye's syndrome, which has occurred less frequently in recent years, has been associated with influenza (and varicella) in patients receiving aspirin, and influenza vaccination may prevent this. Influenza vaccine is not approved for use in infants under 6 months old. No information is available about reactivity, immunogenicity, and adverse reactions in this age group.

347. The answer is e. *(Behrman, 16/e, pp. 848–850. McMillan 3/e, pp. 1006–1009. Rudolph, 20/e, pp. 596–598.)* Clinical manifestations of shigellosis range from watery stools for several days to severe infection with high fever, abdominal pain, and generalized seizures. In general, about 50 percent of these children have emesis, greater than two thirds have fever, 10 percent to 35 percent have seizures, and 40 percent have blood in their stool. Often, the seizure precedes diarrhea and is the complaint that brings the family to the physician. Fever usually lasts about 72 h and the diarrhea resolves within 1 week. Presumptive diagnosis can be made on the clinical history; confirmation is through stool culture. Supportive care, including adequate fluid and electrolyte support, is the mainstay of therapy. Antibiotic treatment is problematic; resistance to trimethoprim-sulfamethoxazole is common, necessitating therapy with third-generation cephalosporins in many cases.

348. The answer is d. *(Behrman, 16/e, pp. 725–727, 803–804. McMillan 3/e, pp. 924–932, 1012–1017. Rudolph, 20/e, pp. 495–497, 604–609.)* Kawasaki syndrome is an acute febrile illness of unknown etiology and shares many of its clinical manifestations with scarlet fever. Scarlatiniform rash, desquamation, erythema of the mucous membranes that produces an injected pharynx and strawberry tongue, and cervical lymphadenopathy are prominent findings in both. The most serious complication of Kawasaki syndrome and scarlet fever is cardiac involvement. Erythrogenic toxin-producing group A β-hemolytic streptococcus is the agent responsible for scarlet fever. Isolation of the organism from the nasopharynx and a rise in antistreptolysin titers will confirm the diagnosis. Serologic tests for a variety of infectious agents, both viral and bacterial, have been negative in Kawasaki syndrome. Rheumatic heart disease is a serious sequela of streptococcal pharyngitis, which can be prevented by appropriate treatment with penicillin. Coronary artery aneurysm and thrombosis are the most serious complications of Kawasaki syndrome. The current approach to treatment, which includes aspirin and IV gamma globulin administered within a week of the onset of fever, appears to lower the prevalence of coronary artery dilatation and aneurysm and shorten the acute phase of the illness.

349. The answer is b. *(Behrman, 16/e, pp. 2037–2038. McMillan 3/e, pp. 1153–1155. Rudolph, 20/e, pp. 933–934.)* *Trichophyton tonsurans* is a major cause of tinea capitis. It produces an infection within the hair follicle that is unresponsive to topical treatment alone and requires long-term therapy with griseofulvin for eradication. Fluorescence is absent on examination by Wood's lamp. Diagnosis is made by microscopic examination of KOH preparation of infected hairs and by culture on appropriate media. A severe form of tinea capitis known as kerion is shown in the photograph. Keep in mind that a diagnosis of tinea capitis and not seborrhea should be considered in any child between the ages of 6 months and puberty who presents with scaliness and hair loss, even if mild. Seborrhea rarely occurs in that age group.

350. The answer is b. (*Behrman, 16/e, pp. 964–966, 1497–1499. McMillan 3/e, pp. 1098–1100. Rudolph, 20/e, pp. 668–669.*) Fifth disease (erythema infectiosum), long recognized as a benign mild exanthem of school-aged children, is now known to be caused by human parvovirus B-19. In the compromised patient, the parvovirus can cause serious anemia by infecting red-cell precursors and causing them to lyse. Patients with hemolytic anemia, such as sickle cell anemia, can develop a transient aplastic crisis. In patients with immunodeficiency, the B-19 infection can be persistent and lead to life-threatening chronic anemia. Infection in a pregnant woman can result in severe anemia in the infected fetus, with secondary hydrops fetalis and death. Roseola is now thought to be caused most often by the human herpesvirus 6. Coxsackie A-16 virus causes hand-foot-mouth disease. Echo-11 virus frequently causes viral meningitis, and cytomegalovirus causes a congenital infection.

351–352. The answers are 351–d, 352–b. (*Behrman, 16/e, pp. 919–920, 1652–1653. McMillan, 3/e, p. 1558. Rudolph, 20/e, p. 76.*) Acute scrotal swelling and pain in a sexually active adolescent should raise the suspicion of epididymitis. Causative organisms are usually gonococci or chlamydiae, but the offending organism is frequently not recovered. Supportive evidence includes pyuria without organisms. Treatment is bed rest, antibiotics, and counseling. The most important differential diagnosis is torsion of the testes.

353. The answer is e. (*Behrman, 16/e, pp. 751–757. McMillan, 3/e, pp. 413–416, 855–883. Rudolph, 20/e, pp. 530–535, 544–548.*) Unsuspected bacteremia due to *Haemophilus influenzae* type b (now rare), *Neisseria menigitidis*, or *Streptococcus pneumoniae* should be considered before prescribing treatment for otitis media in a young, febrile, toxic-appearing infant. Blood culture should be performed before antibiotic therapy is initiated, and examination of the cerebrospinal fluid is indicated if meningitis is suspected. The classic signs of meningitis are found with increasing reliability in children over the age of 6 months. Nevertheless, a febrile, irritable, inconsolable infant with an altered state of alertness deserves a lumbar puncture even in the absence of meningeal signs. A petechial rash, characteristically associated with meningococcal infection, has been known to occur with other bacterial infections as well. Organisms may be identified on smear of these lesions.

A fever accompanied by inability to flex rather than rotate the neck immediately suggests meningitis. An indolent clinical course does not rule out bacterial meningitis. A lumbar puncture is of prime diagnostic importance in determining the presence of bacterial meningitis, which requires immediate antibiotic therapy. A delay in treatment can lead to complications such as cerebrovascular thrombosis, obstructive hydrocephalus, cerebritis with seizures or acute increased intracranial pressure, coma, or death. In the described patient, lumbar puncture is warranted because of the change in his clinical status.

354. The answer is d. *(Behrman, 16/e, pp. 838–842. McMillan, 3/e, pp. 990–993. Rudolph, 20/e, pp. 585–587.)* Newborn infants exposed to pertussis are at considerable risk of being infected regardless of the immune status of the mother. In contrast to other childhood infectious diseases, pertussis is not prevented by transplacentally acquired antibody. Hyperimmune globulin is ineffective and not recommended. Natural immunity conferred by infection is lifelong. Because immunity acquired by immunization declines with age, however, many adults who were immunized in infancy are susceptible to pertussis. Erythromycin achieves high concentrations in respiratory secretions and is effective in eliminating organisms from the respiratory tract of patients. In exposed, susceptible persons, erythromycin may be effective in preventing or lessening severity of the disease if administered during the preparoxysmal stage. Immunization against pertussis is unnecessary if the patient has had culture-proven pertussis.

355. The answer is e. *(Behrman, 16/e, pp. 977–981. McMillan, 3/e, pp. 1107–1110. Rudolph, 20/c, pp. 639–642.)* To prove a diagnosis of infectious mononucleosis, a triad of findings should be present. First, physical findings can include diffuse adenopathy, tonsillar enlargement, an enlarged spleen, small hemorrhages on the soft palate, and periorbital swelling. Second, the hematologic changes should reveal a predominance of lymphocytes with at least 10 percent of these cells being atypical. Third, the characteristic antibody response should be present. Traditionally, heterophil antibodies can be detected when confirming a diagnosis of infectious mononucleosis. These antibodies may not be present, however, particularly in young children. Alternatively, specific antibodies against viral antigens on the Epstein-Barr virus can be measured. Antibodies to viral capsid antigen (VCA) and to anti-D early antigen are elevated prior to the appearance of

Epstein-Barr nuclear antigen (EBNA) and are, therefore, markers for acute infection. IgG VCA and EBNA persist for life, whereas anti-D disappears after 6 months.

356. The answer is b. (*Behrman, 16/e, pp. 776–780. McMillan, 3/e, pp. 1009–1012, 2127–2128. Rudolph, 20/e, pp. 548–551, 602.*) Acute osteomyelitis tends to begin abruptly with fever and marked, localized bone tenderness that usually occurs at the metaphysis. Redness and swelling frequently follow. Although usually the result of hematogenous bacterial spread, particularly of *Staphylococcus aureus*, acute osteomyelitis can follow an episode of deep cellulitis and should be suspected whenever deep cellulitis occurs. Diagnosis must often be based on clinical grounds because bone changes may not be visible on x-ray for up to 12 days after onset of the disease. Bone scans with radionuclides, however, can be useful in the early diagnosis of osteomyelitis and in its differentiation from cellulitis and septic arthritis. Caution must be exercised, however, when interpreting a normal bone scan in a patient suspected of having osteomyelitis; falsely normal bone scans do occur in patients with active bone infection. Antibiotic treatment must be initiated immediately to avoid further extension of infection into bone, where adequate drug levels are difficult to achieve. Treatment is usually continued for at least 3 weeks.

357. The answer is c. (*Behrman, 16/e, pp. 810–813. McMillan, 3/e, pp. 404–413, 421–427. Rudolph, 20/e, pp. 536–548.*) Many organisms can cause meningitis in the neonate including *Escherichia coli, Listeria, Haemophilus influenzae,* gram-negative rods, group B streptococci, and coagulase-positive and coagulase-negative staphylococci. Clinical manifestations of meningitis in neonates include lethargy, bulging fontanelle, seizures, and nuchal rigidity. The diagnosis is made with examination and culture of the cerebrospinal fluid. Treatment is begun while awaiting the results of the spinal fluid analysis. Appropriate antibiotic coverage must include activity against gram-positive and gram-negative organisms (ampicillin and gentamicin or cefotaxime).

358. The answer is c. (*Behrman, 16/e, pp. 875–878. McMillan, 3/e, pp. 940–942, 1969–1970. Rudolph, 20/e, pp. 555–558.*) Infant botulism is a neuromuscular disease caused by the toxin of *Clostridium botulinum*. The disease is distinct from classic botulism in that spores are ingested and the toxin is synthesized by the organism while it resides in the infant's intestine. The toxin is then absorbed and produces weakness and paralysis because of impaired release of acetylcholine at the neuromuscular synapse. Recent evidence suggests a broad clinical spectrum of infant botulism. Some infants may never require hospitalization and demonstrate only minimal feeding difficulties. More severely affected infants can have a presentation that suggests the sudden infant death syndrome. Infants who survive show a complete resolution of symptoms.

359. The answer is a. *(Behrman, 16/e, pp. 743, 803. McMillan, 3/e, pp. 850–855, 961–964, 995–998, 1002–1006, 1124–1126. Rudolph, 20/e, pp. 530–536, 567–570, 594–595, 654–655.)* In an infant who appears otherwise normal, the sudden onset of high fever together with a marked elevation and shift to the left of the white blood cell count suggests pneumococcal bacteremia. Viral infections such as roseola seldom cause such profound shifts in the blood leukocyte count. Streptococcosis refers to prolonged, low-grade, insidious nasopharyngitis that sometimes occurs in infants infected with group A β-hemolytic streptococci. Neither typhoid fever nor diphtheria produces markedly high white blood cell counts; both are characterized by headache, malaise, and other systemic signs. Other bacteria that should be considered in a child with this presentation include *Haemophilus influenzae* type b and meningococcus.

360. The answer is c. *(Behrman, 16/e, pp. 951–953. McMillan, 3/e, pp. 442–444, 1135–1136. Rudolph, 20/e, pp. 681–683.)* When German measles (rubella) occurs during the first 2 months of pregnancy, it has a severe effect on the fetus, including cardiac defects, cataracts, and glaucoma. The most common cardiac defects are patent ductus arteriosus, which can be accompanied by peripheral pulmonary artery stenosis and atrial and ventricular septal defects. Myriad other complications vary in incidence with the timing of the infection during pregnancy, including thrombocytopenia, hepatosplenomegaly, hepatitis, hemolytic anemia, microcephaly, and a higher risk of developing insulin-dependent diabetes mellitus.

361. The answer is d. *(Behrman, 16/e, pp. 836, 1934-1935. McMillan, 3/e, p. 670. Rudolph, 20/e, pp. 2118–2119.)* The presence of proptosis, pain, edema of the conjunctiva, ophthalmoplegia, and a decrease or loss of visual acuity distinguishes orbital cellulitis from periorbital or preseptal cellulitis. In the latter condition, the globe has a full range of motion and vision is unimpaired. The most common cause of orbital cellulitis in children is infection in the adjacent paranasal sinuses. Computed tomography (CT) scan of the orbit is indicated to determine the extent of orbital involvement and the need for surgical intervention for drainage of infected sinuses, orbital abscesses, or subperiosteal abscesses.

362. The answer is d. *(Behrman, 16/e, pp. 946–950. McMillan, 3/e, pp. 1137–1141. Rudolph, 20/e, pp. 661–666.)* The picture and clinical history presented are most common for the diagnosis of measles (roseola). This is an uncommon disease in areas where immunization rates are high, but sporadic outbreaks do occur. The rash typically lasts 6 days. Complications are common including pneumonia, laryngitis, myocarditis, and encephalitis.

363. The answer is a. *(Behrman, 16/e, pp. 1275–1278. McMillan, 3/e, pp. 572, 971, 997, 1307–1310. Rudolph, 20/e, pp. 573–580, 674–676, 1633–1634.)* Children who have acute epiglottitis, a life-threatening infection of the hypopharynx and epiglottis caused by *Haemophilus influenzae*, typically present with high fever, extremely sore throat, and a croupy cough. It is now a rare disease due to the widespread use of Hib vaccine. An increased incidence of epiglottitis is now seen due to *Streptococcus pneumoniae* and in immunocompromised children. Physical examination characteristically shows a red throat and a red, swollen epiglottis that can be obscured by exudate or so distorted that its identity is misinterpreted. It is important that caution be exercised while attempting to visualize the epiglottis. Abrupt glottic spasm is a well-recognized, potentially fatal complication in these patients. Affected children often are unable to swallow saliva, and because the swollen epiglottis can unpredictably and suddenly cause total and fatal airway obstruction, immediate hospitalization is mandatory, even in the absence of severe respiratory distress. If a diagnosis of acute epiglottitis is uncertain, a lateral x-ray of the neck will differentiate epiglottic from subglottic swelling, the latter being associated with a less serious disease, viral croup.

364. The answer is a. *(Behrman, 16/e, 946–953, 964–966, 984–986, 1989–1990. McMillan, 3/e, pp. 721–722, 1098–1100; 1124–1125, 1134–1140. Rudolph, 20/e, pp. 654–655, 661–666, 668–669, 679–681, 907.)* Symptoms of rubella, usually a mild disease, include a diffuse maculopapular rash that lasts for 3 days, marked enlargement of the posterior cervical and occipital lymph nodes, low-grade fever, mild sore throat, and, occasionally, conjunctivitis, arthralgia, or arthritis. Persons with rubeola develop a severe cough, coryza, photophobia, conjunctivitis, and a high fever that reaches its peak at the height of the generalized macular rash, which typically lasts for 5 days. Koplik's spots on the buccal mucosa are diagnostic. Roseola is a viral exanthem of infants in which the high fever abruptly abates as a rash appears. Erythema infectiosum (fifth disease) begins with bright erythema on the cheeks ("slapped cheek" sign), followed by a red maculopapular rash on the trunk and extremities, which fades centrally at first. Erythema multiforme is a poorly understood syndrome consisting of skin lesions and involvement of mucous membranes. A number of infectious agents and drugs have been associated with this syndrome.

365. The answer is c. *(Behrman, 16/e, pp. 954–955. McMillan, 3/e, pp. 1141–1142. Rudolph, 20/e, pp. 666–668.)* Although mumps is usually thought of as a parotitis, it is a generalized infection and, as such, can have widespread effects and a variety of clinical presentations. Many infections with the mumps virus are unrecognized because of the substantial rate of subclinical attacks. Meningitis, pancreatitis, and renal involvement can occur as part of the disease. The meningitis that occurs with mumps can occur at the same time as the parotitis, or following the parotitis by about 10 days. Orchitis, seen most frequently in postpubertal males, has been reported in young children as well. All of these problems can be prevented by prior immunization with live attenuated virus vaccine. Many patients with mumps have some white cells in their spinal fluid. Arthritis is rare in children. Subendocardial fibroelastosis in a newborn was once thought to be associated with prenatal infection with mumps, but this does not appear to be true.

366. The answer is c. *(Behrman, 16/e, pp. 769–771. McMillan, 3/e, pp. 447–448, 1723–1725. Rudolph, 20/e, pp. 647–651.)* Hepatitis A (infectious hepatitis) is characterized by a relatively short incubation period (15 to 50 days) following transmission of the virus, which is primarily by the fecal-oral route. Its onset is abrupt, with sudden fever, nausea, vomiting, anorexia, and tenderness of the liver, soon followed by jaundice. Subclinical infections are common. Elevated serum levels of bilirubin and aspartate aminotransferase (glutamic oxaloacetic transaminase, SGOT) are transient, usually not persisting for more than 3 weeks. Viremia is brief and the period of maximum infectivity of stools usually occurs during the 2 weeks prior to the onset of jaundice. Hepatitis B (serum hepatitis), usually transmitted parenterally via blood or blood products, can also be transmitted nonparenterally via body fluids such as saliva or semen. Following a long incubation period (40 to 180 days), there is a gradual onset of low fever, anorexia, and jaundice, often preceded or accompanied by extrahepatic manifestations such as macular rashes, arthralgias, or urticaria, which may mimic serum sickness. Levels of SGOT and serum bilirubin can be elevated for months, the latter sometimes rising to levels greater than 20 mg/dL when associated with the fulminant hepatitis more often seen with hepatitis B infection. Viremia usually persists throughout the clinical course of hepatitis B infections and can progress to a chronic carrier state in 10 percent of affected persons, most of whom are asymptomatic. These can be identified by the persistence of the viral surface antigen HBsAg in their blood. A third type of hepatitis, hepatitis C (formerly known as non-A, non-B hepatitis), is important because it accounts for 80 percent to 90 percent of posttransfusion hepatitis in the United States. In addition, it is associated with a high rate of chronicity (25 percent to 50 percent).

367. The answer is a. (*Behrman, 16/e, pp. 1800–1801. McMillan, 3/e, pp. 2267–2268.*) The importance and urgency of the lumbar puncture in cases of suspected meningitis outweigh the usual niceties in the performance of procedures. Infants and children require adequate restraints, preferably local anesthesia, and sometimes, sedation. Contraindications are few and include increased intracranial pressure in the patient without an open fontanelle that can result in herniation, severe cardiorespiratory distress, skin infection at the puncture site, and severe thrombocytopenia.

368. The answer is e. (*Behrman, 16/e, pp. 797–798, 865–867, 910–914, 922–925. McMillan, 3/e, pp. 717–718, 898–902, 951–953, 1012, 1017–1021, 1137–1140, 2160–2162. Rudolph, 20/e, pp. 582–583, 626–628, 689–692, 2010–2011.*) The incubation period for Rocky Mountain spotted fever (RMSF) has a range of 1 to 14 days. A brief prodromal period consisting of headache and malaise is typically followed by the abrupt onset of fever and chills. A maculopapular rash starts on the second to fourth day of illness on the flexor surfaces of the wrists and ankles before moving in a central direction. Typically, the palms and soles are involved. The rash can become hemorrhagic within 1 or 2 days. Hyponatremia and thrombocytopenia may be seen.

Tuleramia has a variable presentation including abrupt onset of fever, chills, malaise, weakness, and headache, and also a variety of skin rashes. Children often have fever, pharyngitis, hepatosplenomegaly, and non-specific constitutional symptoms.

In the differential diagnosis of RMSF are a number of other diseases. A morbilliform eruption can precede a petechial rash caused by *Neisseria meningitidis*. Viral infections, particularly by the enteroviruses, can cause a severe illness that resembles RMSF. Atypical measles is seen primarily in persons who received the killed measles vaccine before 1968. After exposure to wild-type measles, such a person can develop a prodrome consisting of fever, cough, headache, and myalgia. This is usually followed by the development of pneumonia and an urticarial rash beginning on the extremities. Toxic shock syndrome (TSS) is a disease characterized by sudden onset of fever, diarrhea, shock, inflammation of mucous membranes, and a diffuse macular rash resulting in desquamation of the hands and feet. Lyme disease is seen with an early period of localized disease including erythema migrans, possibly with flu-like symptoms, followed by a distinctive period of erythema migrans, arthralgia, arthritis, meningitis, neuritis, and carditis.

369. The answer is e. *(Behrman, 16/e, pp. 885–897. McMillan, 3/e, pp. 1026–1039. Rudolph, 20/e, pp. 614–616.)* Allergic response to tubercle bacilli is the basis for the intracutaneous Mantoux test for tuberculosis; the test becomes positive within 2 to 10 weeks after infection. Cross-reactions to atypical mycobacteria sometimes occur. The Mantoux test can become negative during advanced stages of tuberculosis or briefly after immunization with live virus vaccines (such as those for measles, mumps, and rubella) and administration of corticosteroids or immunosuppressive drugs; otherwise it is positive for life. A positive skin test in a child likely warrants antimicrobial therapy. Children, who rarely develop cavitary disease, are not contagious.

370. The answer is c. *(Behrman, 16/e, p. 1990. McMillan, 3/e, pp. 721–722. Rudolph, 20/e, p. 907.)* The combination of erythema multiforme and vesicular, ulcerated lesions of the mucous membranes of the eyes, mouth, anus, and urethra defines the Stevens-Johnson syndrome. Fever is common and even pulmonary involvement occasionally is noted; the mortality can approach 10 percent. Common complications include corneal ulceration, dehydration due to severe stomatitis, and subsequently, poor fluid intake, and urinary retention caused by dysuria. Among the known causes of the Stevens-Johnson syndrome are allergy to various drugs (including phenytoin, barbiturates, sulfonamides, and penicillin) and infection with a variety of organisms including *Mycoplasma pneumoniae* or herpes type 1.

371. The answer is e. *(Behrman, 16/e, pp. 944–945, 1036–1040, 1067–1068, 1072–1073. McMillan, 3/e, pp. 1164–1166, 1174–1177, 1193–1195, 1198–1203. Rudolph, 20/e, pp. 710–712, 714–720, 725–726, 734–736.)* Many common parasites travel through body tissue to create disease. *Ascaris lumbricoides* larvae travel through the intestinal wall and end up, by way of the liver, in the lungs, where they commonly produce pneumonia and peripheral eosinophilia (Löffler's syndrome); worms mature in the small intestine, where they sometimes cause obstruction. The larvae of *Toxocara canis* migrate from the intestine to all parts of the body, where granulomatous reactions can occur (visceral larva migrans). Hookworms (*Necator americanus*) can cause intestinal blood loss from mucosal laceration; cutaneous larva migrans occurs when hookworm larvae fail to enter cutaneous blood vessels after penetrating the skin. Following the ingestion of pork or other improperly cooked meat infected with *Trichinella spiralis*, the parasites penetrate the gut wall and migrate to striated muscle and, occasionally, to heart and CNS, where they become encysted and remain viable for years. *Enterobius vermicularis* (pinworm) causes a localized infestation and does not have a tissue phase. Sporotrichosis is a chronic fungal infection that typically is limited to cutaneous and subcutaneous tissues. *Giardia* and *Cryptosporidium* rarely penetrate the gut wall, instead causing gas, diarrhea, and bloating as common findings.

372. The answer is c. *(Behrman, 16/e, pp. 910–914. McMillan, 3/e, pp. 951–953, 2160–2162. Rudolph, 20/e, pp. 582–583.)* Lyme disease, caused by the spirochete *Borrelia burgdorferi* and transmitted mostly by ticks of the ioxodes family, is characterized by a unique skin lesion, recurrent attacks of arthritis, and occasional involvement of the heart and central nervous system. Illness usually appears in late summer or early fall, 2 to 30 days after a bite by an infecting tick. Erythema chronicum migrans begins as a red macule, usually on the trunk at the site of tick attachment that enlarges in a circular fashion with central clearing. Nonspecific systemic signs include headache, fever, and malaise. Joint involvement generally occurs days to years after onset of the rash. Cardiac disease consists primarily of disturbances of rhythm. Involvement of the central nervous system is evidenced by headache and stiff neck. The diagnosis should be suspected when any of the signs and symptoms occur because the disease can present in an atypical manner. The characteristic lesion of erythema chronicum migrans as well as the history of tick bite have frequently not been noted by the patient. It is not until late joint, heart, or neurologic manifestations occur, and Lyme disease is suspected, that serologic evidence confirms the etiology. Serologic evidence is sought when the patient has spent time in summer months in endemic areas or there is a risk of tick bite. Treatment with penicillin or tetracycline results in a faster resolution of symptoms and prevention of later complications, especially if given early in the course of the disease.

373. The answer is e. *(Behrman, 16/e, pp. 826–828. McMillan, 3/e, pp. 982, 901. Rudolph, 20/e, pp. 691 692, 2010–2011.)* Rocky Mountain spotted fever and meningococcemia can present in a similar fashion. Meningococcemia can be complicated by a variety of disorders, including meningitis, purulent pericarditis, endocarditis, pneumonia, otitis media, and arthritis. (Arthritis associated with meningococcemia may be mediated by an immune mechanism rather than bacterial invasion of the joint.) The potent endotoxin of the causative organism, *Neisseria meningitidis*, can induce shock, disseminated intravascular coagulation with associated hemorrhaging, and acute adrenal failure caused by localized intraadrenal bleeding; these reactions can be collectively referred to as the Waterhouse-Friderichsen syndrome. Vaccines against *N. meningitidis* groups A, C, Y, and W135 are now available. Prophylaxis with sulfadiazine for sensitive organisms or with rifampin for those in close contact with affected persons is recommended. In contrast, Rocky Mountain spotted fever is often a more indolent infection with a rash developing days after the onset of the fever and other symptoms. This course is not invariable, however, and antibiotic therapy for the patient for whom Rocky Mountain spotted fever and meningococcemia cannot be differentiated should not be delayed.

374. The answer is c. *(Behrman, 16/e, 1277–1278. McMillan, 3/e, pp. 1307–1310. Rudolph, 20/e, pp. 1633–1634.)* Croup involves the larynx and trachea; it usually is caused by parainfluenza or respiratory syncytial viruses.

The usual age range for presentation is 6 months to 6 years. Symptoms include low-grade fever, barking cough, and hoarse, inspiratory stridor without wheezing. The pharynx can be normal or slightly red, and the lungs usually clear. In children in severe respiratory distress, prolonged dyspnea can progress to physical exhaustion and fatal respiratory failure. Because agitation can be a sign of hypoxia, sedation should not be ordered. Hyperinflation on chest x-ray is seen in asthma, not croup.

375. The answer is e. *(Behrman, 16/e, pp. 842–848, 944–945, 1039–1040, 1054–1062, 1067–1068. McMillan, 3/e, pp. 1002–1006, 1164–1166, 1174–1176, 1184–1193, 1995. Rudolph, 20/e, pp. 592–596, 710–712, 717–719, 772–775.)* *Cryptosporidium* has become an important cause of diarrhea in immunocompromised patients, particularly those with AIDS. It can also affect patients who are immunocompetent, and with increased experience in the laboratory detection of the organism, it has been recognized as an agent responsible for epidemics of diarrhea in day care centers. Persistent, nonsuppurative diarrhea can be caused by such organisms as amebas, whipworms (trichuriasis), *cryptosporidium*, or *Giardia lamblia*. *Salmonella sonnei* can be grown in culture, but microscopy is not helpful other than finding fecal leukocytes. *Enterobius vermicularis* is pinworms, which causes rectal itching and not diarrhea. Sporotrichosis is a fungal infection of the cutaneous and subcutaneous tissue that typically does not cause diarrhea. Acquired *Toxoplasma gondii* can infest any body tissue. Infection can result in fever, myalgia, lymphadenopathy, maculopapular rash, hepatomegaly, pneumonia, encephalitis, chorioretinitis, or myocarditis. This intracellular parasite does not ordinarily cause diarrhea and is not found in stools. Congenital toxoplasmosis can occur if a mother first acquires the parasite during pregnancy. Her infected newborn infant can demonstrate jaundice, hepatosplenomegaly, hydrocephalus or microcephaly, intracranial calcification, or chorioretinitis.

376–379. The answers are 376–b, 377–a, 378–e, 379–c. *(Behrman, 16/e, pp. 331, 595–597, 599–600, 602–604. McMillan, 3/e, pp. 867, 2071–2072, 2092–2101. Rudolph, 20/e, pp. 437–441, 444, 446–449.)* Many primary immunologic deficiencies can be classified as defects of T-lymphocyte function (containment of fungi, protozoa, acid-fast bacteria, and certain viruses) and B-lymphocyte function (synthesis and secretion of immunoglobulins). Among the T-cell diseases is DiGeorge anomaly, in which defective embryologic development of the third and fourth pharyngeal pouches results in hypoplasia of both thymus and parathyroid glands. Associated findings with DiGeorge anomaly include CATCH: C for cardiac, A for abnormal faces, T for thymic hypoplasia, C for cleft palate, and H for hypocalcemia.

Primary B-cell diseases include panhypogammaglobulinemia (Bruton's disease), an X-linked deficiency of all three major classes of immunoglobulins, as well as other selective deficiencies of the immunoglobulins or their subgroups.

Combined T- and B-cell diseases include the X-linked recessive Wiskott-Aldrich syndrome of mild T-cell dysfunction, diminished serum IgM, marked elevation of IgA and IgE, eczema, recurrent middle ear infections, lymphopenia, and thrombocytopenia. Patients with the catastrophic combined T- and B-cell disease, known as severe combined immunodeficiency disease (Swiss-type lymphopenic agammaglobulinemia or SCID), have deficient T- and B-cells. Consequently, they are both marked lymphopenia and agammaglobulinemia, as well as hypoplasia of the thymus. Chronic diarrhea; rashes; recurrent, serious bacterial, fungal, or viral infections; wasting; and early death are characteristic. Other T- and B-cell deficiencies include ataxia-telangiectasia and chronic mucocutaneous candidiasis

Job-Buckley syndrome is a disorder of phagocytic chemotaxis associated with hypergammaglobulin E, eczema-like rash, and recurrent severe staphylococcal infections.

380–385. The answers are 380–b, 381–b, 382–a, 383–d, 384–b, 385–f. *(Behrman, 16/e, pp. 862–864, 872–873, 984–986, 1147–1150, 1315–1317. McMillan, 3/e, pp. 956–961, 998–1101, 1124–1125. Rudolph, 20/e, pp. 560–562, 664–665, 865, 1089–1091, 1640–1641.)* The evidence is mounting that *Rochalimaea henselae* is the major etiologic agent for cat-scratch disease. History of a scratch or a bite of a kitten is often positive and fleas are often a factor in transmission. Diagnosis is usually by history and presenting signs and symptoms.

Infection with *Helicobacter pylori* is associated with antral gastritis and primary duodenal ulcer disease. Culture for *H. pylori* requires endoscopy and gastric biopsy. The biopsied tissue can be tested for urease activity and examined histologically after special staining. Alternatively, noninvasive tests involving detection of metabolic products of *H. pylori* (urease activity) or antibodies against *H. pylori* can be demonstrated.

Roseola (exanthema subitum) is a common acute illness of young children, characterized by several days of high fever followed by a rapid defervescence and the appearance of an evanescent, erythematous, maculo-papular rash. Human herpesvirus 6 (HHV) has been identified as its main cause.

Pseudomonas is a ubiquitous organism. Most infections with the organism are opportunistic, involving several organs. Skin infections related to burns, trauma (such as in a puncture wound through a tennis shoe), and use of swimming pools are not uncommon. Injuries through a tennis shoe are prone to pseudomonal infections due to the warm, moist nature of the shoe's environment. In contrast, a wound through a bare foot would be associated with cutaneous flora such as *Staphylococcus*. Cystic fibrosis is characterized by a predilection for colonization of airways with *Staphylococcus aureus* and *Pseudomonas aeruginosa*. *Pseudomonas cepacia* infection is not as common, but it is more problematic.

386–388. The answers are 386–b, 387–a, 388–d. *(Behrman, 16/e, pp. 1067–1068, 1967. McMillan, 3/e, pp. 918, 1153–1155, 1195. Rudolph, 20/e, pp. 717–719, 882–883.)* Several simple tests are available to assist in the diagnosis of dermatologic conditions. Among these are the Wood's lamp, which uses a wavelength of 365 nm to identify fungal infections of the skin. Blue-green fluorescence is detected at the base of hair shafts infected with certain strains of fungus responsible for tinea capitis. A negative Wood's lamp result does not rule out fungal infection because not all strains become apparent.

For a Tzanck smear, the base of a freshly ruptured blister is scraped, stained with Giemsa stain, and examined under the microscope. Some viral infections such as herpes and varicella will demonstrate balloon cells and multinucleated giant cells.

Pinworms (*Enterobius vermicularis*) lay their eggs at night on the perianal region. These eggs can be gathered by pressing cellophane tape to the perianal region at night or early in the morning. This tape is then examined under the microscope to detect the characteristic eggs.

389–392. The answers are 389–c, 390–a, 391–g, 392–e. *(Behrman, 16/e, pp. 761–765, 885–897, 914–921. McMillan, 3/e, pp. 451–452, 893–894, 897, 1009–1012, 1026–1039, 1217, 1227–1230. Rudolph, 20/e, pp. 602, 614–623, 686–688, 1654–1655.)* Approximately 10 percent to 20 percent of infants born to mothers with *Chlamydia trachomatis* infection develop pneumonia. The presentation of this pneumonia usually occurs between 1 and 3 months of age with cough, tachypnea, and lack of fever. Examination reveals rales but not wheezing. Laboratory data suggestive of *C. trachomatis* infection include an increase in eosinophils in the peripheral blood. The chest radiograph shows hyperinflation with interstitial infiltrates.

Mycoplasma pneumoniae is a common cause of pneumonia in the school-aged child or the young adult. Usual presentation includes the gradual onset of headache, malaise, fever, and lower respiratory symptoms. Typically, the cough (often nonproductive) worsens for the first 2 weeks of the illness then slowly resolves over the ensuing 3 to 4 weeks. Early in the disease, the physical examination is remarkable for a paucity of signs; the patient usually has a few fine rales. Later, the dyspnea and fever become worse. Radiographic findings include an interstitial or bronchial pattern, especially in the lower lobes, and commonly only on one side. The diagnosis is usually made on clinical grounds.

Staphylococcal pneumonia is caused by *S. aureus*. It is a rapidly progressive and life-threatening form of pneumonia most commonly seen in children less than 1 year of age. Commonly, the child has an upper respiratory infection for several days with the abrupt onset of fever and respiratory distress. Pleural effusion, empyema, and pyopneumothorax are common complications. Laboratory evidence of this disease can include a markedly elevated WBC count with left shift. Radiographic findings include nonspecific bronchopneumonia early in the disease, which later becomes more dense and homogeneous and involves an entire lobe or hemithorax.

A high index of suspicion is helpful to diagnose tuberculosis. Tuberculosis should be considered in any patient with pneumonia who belongs to a high-risk group, including poor and indigent persons, present and former residents of correctional institutions, homeless persons, IV drug abusers, health care workers caring for high-risk patients, and children exposed to high-risk adults. Clinical and radiographic findings are variable in children, but include nonspecific cough and dyspnea. Radiographic findings often include hilar adenopathy, focal hyperinflation, and atelectasis.

HEMATOLOGIC AND NEOPLASTIC DISEASES

Questions

DIRECTIONS: Each item below contains a question or incomplete statement followed by suggested responses. Select the **one best** response to each question.

Items 393–394

393. Two weeks after a viral syndrome a 2-year-old child develops bruising and generalized petechiae, more prominent over the legs. No hepatosplenomegaly or lymph node enlargement is noted. The examination is otherwise unremarkable. Laboratory testing shows the patient to have a normal hemoglobin, hematocrit, and white blood count and differential. The platelet count is 15,000/mm^3. The most likely diagnosis is

a. von Willebrand's disease
b. acute leukemia
c. idiopathic (immune) thrombocytopenic purpura
d. aplastic anemia
e. thrombotic thrombocytopenic purpura

394. Appropriate treatment of this child includes

a. intravenous gamma globulin
b. platelet transfusion
c. aspirin therapy
d. factor VIII infusion
e. prednisone, vincristine, and asparaginase induction followed by methotrexate and 6-mercaptopurine

395. Which of the following is commonly associated with thrombocytopenia in the newborn?

a. congenital cytomegalovirus infection
b. uncomplicated prematurity
c. chlamydial conjunctivitis
d. maternal ingestion of aspirin
e. nasolacrimal duct stenosis

396. An increased concentration of hemoglobin A_2 is found in children with

a.   iron deficiency
b. β-thalassemia trait
c.   sickle cell anemia
d.   chronic systemic illness
e.   lead poisoning

397. A 3-year-old child presents with a petechial rash but is otherwise well and without physical findings. Platelet count is 20,000/mm^3; hemoglobin and WBC count are normal. The most likely diagnosis is

a.   immune thrombocytopenic purpura (ITP)
b.   Henoch-Schönlein purpura
c.   disseminated intravascular coagulopathy (DIC)
d.   acute lymphoblastic leukemia
e.   systemic lupus erythematosus (SLE)

398. 4-year-old previously well boy develops pallor, dark urine, and jaundice. There has been no apparent exposure to a jaundiced person or to any toxins. He is taking trimethoprim-sulfamethoxazole for otitis media. You consider the possibility of a hemolytic crisis caused by glucose-6-phosphate dehydrogenase (G6PD) deficiency. In which of the following ethnic groups is the incidence LOWEST?

a.   African-American
b.   Greek
c.   Chinese
d.   Middle Eastern
e.   Scandinavian

399. Mass neonatal screening for hemoglobinopathy has made it possible to institute comprehensive care in very early infancy. In the United States, the incidence of SS, SC, and S β-thalassemia combined is 1:400. Special precautionary measures for newborns with a hemoglobinopathy include which of the following?

a.   monthly injections of vitamin B_{12}
b.   tetracycline
c.   meningococcal vaccine in early childhood
d.   education of parents regarding abdominal palpation and temperature taking
e.   every 6 week infusion of immunoglobulin

400. A 2950-g black baby boy is born at home at term. On arrival at the hospital, he appears pale, but the physical examination is otherwise normal. Laboratory studies reveal the following: mother's blood type A, Rh-positive; baby's blood type O, Rh-positive; hematocrit 38; reticulocyte count 5 percent. Which of the following is the most likely cause of the anemia?

a.   fetomaternal transfusion
b.   ABO incompatibility
c.   physiologic anemia of the newborn
d.   sickle cell anemia
e.   iron-deficiency anemia

401. Poor prognostic signs in acute lymphoblastic leukemia include which of the following?

a. presence of a mediastinal mass
b. hyperdiploidy with more than 50 chromosomes
c. white blood cell count at diagnosis of less than 100,000/mm^3
d. age between 1 and 10 years
e. early pre-B-cell variety of the disease

402. While bathing her 2-year-old son, a mother feels a mass in his abdomen. A thorough medical evaluation of the child reveals aniridia, hypospadias, horseshoe kidney, and hemihypertrophy. The most likely diagnosis for this child is

a. neuroblastoma
b. Wilms' tumor
c. hepatoblastoma
d. rhabdomyosarcoma
e. testicular cancer

---

403. A 2-year-old child in shock has multiple non-blanching purple lesions of various sizes scattered about on trunk and extremities; petechiae are noted, and oozing from the puncture site has been observed. The child's peripheral blood smear is presented. Clotting studies are likely to show which of the following?

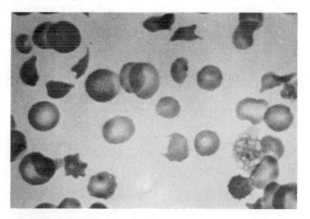

a. increased levels of factor V and VIII
b. a decreased prothrombin level
c. an increased fibrinogen level
d. the presence of fibrin split products
e. normal partial thromboplastin time (PTT)

404. Which of the following most commonly carries increased eosinophilia in the peripheral blood smear?

a.   bacterial infections
b.   chronic allergic rhinitis
c.   fungal infections
d.   helminth infestation
e.   tuberculosis

405. A preterm black male infant was found to be jaundiced 12 h after birth. At 36 h of age, his serum bilirubin was 18 mg/dL, hemoglobin concentration was 12.5 g/dL, and reticulocyte count 9 percent. Many nucleated red cells and some spherocytes were seen in the peripheral blood smear. The differential diagnosis should include which of the following?

a.   pyruvate kinase deficiency
b.   hereditary spherocytosis
c.   sickle cell anemia
d.   Rh incompatibility
e.   polycythemia

Items 406–407

406. On a routine well-child examination, a 1-year-old boy is noted to be pale. He is in the 75th percentile for weight, and the 25th percentile for length. Results of physical examination are otherwise normal. His hematocrit is 24 percent.

Of the following questions, which is most likely to be helpful in making a diagnosis?

a.   What is the child's usual daily diet?
b.   Did the child receive phototherapy for neonatal jaundice?
c.   Has anyone in the family received a blood transfusion?
d.   Is the child on any medications?
e.   What is the pattern and appearance of his bowel movements?

407. Having performed a complete history and physical examination on the patient, you proceed with a diagnostic workup. Initial laboratory results are as follows: hemoglobin 8 g/dL; hematocrit 24 percent; leukocyte count 11,000/mm³ with 38 percent neutrophils, 7 percent bands, 55 percent lymphocytes; hypochromia on smear; free erythrocyte protoporphyrin (FEP) 110 micrograms/dL; lead level 7 micrograms/dL whole blood; platelet count adequate; reticulocyte count 0.5 percent; sickle cell preparation negative; stool guaiac negative; and mean corpuscular volume (MCV) 65 fl. You would most appropriately recommend

a. blood transfusion
b. oral ferrous sulfate
c. intramuscular iron dextran
d. an iron-fortified cereal
e. calcium EDTA

408. A 10-year-old boy is admitted to the hospital because of bleeding. Pertinent laboratory findings include a platelet count of 50,000/mm³, prothrombin time (PT) of 15 sec (control 11.5 sec), activated partial thromboplastin time (aPTT) of 51 sec (control 36 sec), thrombin time (TT) of 13.7 sec (control 10.5 sec), and factor VIII level of 14 percent (normal 38 percent to 178 percent). The most likely cause of his bleeding is

a. immune thrombocytopenic purpura (ITP)
b. vitamin K deficiency
c. disseminated intravascular coagulation (DIC)
d. hemophilia A
e. hemophilia B

409. Which of the following statements concerning important toxicities of antineoplastic agents is true?

a. vincristine can cause hemorrhagic cystitis
b. prednisone can cause alopecia
c. methotrexate can cause GI mucositis
d. 6-mercaptopurine can cause hearing toxicity
e. doxorubicin (Adriamycin) can cause pulmonary fibrosis

410. Which of the following statements regarding Hodgkin's disease is true?

a. Hodgkin's disease in developed countries is more common before the age of 5 years and is rarely seen in adolescents
b. systemic symptoms are rarely seen (less than 5 percent)
c. elevated blast cells in peripheral smears are common
d. in most patients with Hodgkin's disease, the initial mode of spread occurs via lymphatic channels to contiguous lymph nodes
e. staging laparotomy is mandatory in every patient with Hodgkin's disease

---

411. In a seemingly healthy child, the polymorphonuclear neutrophil shown in the following illustration is most likely to be associated with

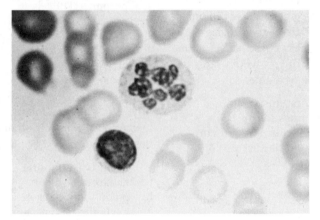

a. malignancy
b. iron deficiency
c. folic acid deficiency
d. Döhle's inclusion bodies
e. the Pelger-Huët nuclear anomaly

DIRECTIONS: Each group of questions below consists of lettered options followed by numbered items. For each numbered item, select the appropriate lettered option(s). Each lettered option may be used once, more than once, or not at all. **Choose exactly the number of options indicated following each item.**

Items 412–415

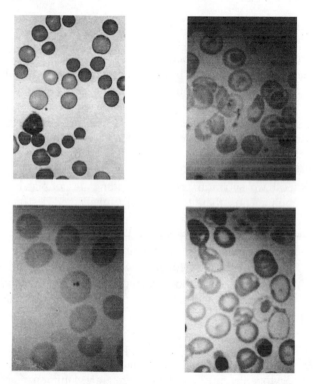

For each disorder listed below, select the peripheral blood smear with which it is most likely to be associated.

412. Howell-Jolly bodies in splenectomized child **(SELECT 1 SMEAR)**

413. Thalassemia major **(SELECT 1 SMEAR)**

414. Hereditary spherocytosis **(SELECT 1 SMEAR)**

415. Hemoglobin C disease **(SELECT 1 SMEAR)**

HEMATOLOGIC AND NEOPLASTIC DISEASES

Answers

393–394. The answers are 393–c, 394–a. *(Behrman, 16/e, pp. 1520–1522. McMillan, 3/e, pp. 367, 1477–1479. Rudolph, 20/e, pp. 1241–1242.)* In children, idiopathic or immune thrombocytopenic purpura (ITP) is the most common form of thrombocytopenic purpura. In most cases a preceding viral infection can be noted. No diagnostic test exists for this disease; exclusion of the other diseases listed in the question is necessary. In this disease, the platelet count is frequently less than 20,000, but other laboratory tests yield essentially normal results, including the bone marrow aspiration (if done). For ITP, platelets are sequestered and destroyed at the spleen by the reticuloendothelial system (RES) that binds self-immunoglobulins attached to the platelet. Exogenous IV gamma globulin can work to saturate the RES binding sites for platelet bound self-immunoglobulin. Thus, there is less platelet uptake and destruction by the spleen.

Aplastic anemia is unlikely if the other cell lines are normal. Von Willebrand's disease might be expected to present with bleeding and not just bruising. It is unlikely that acute leukemia would present with thrombocytopenia only. Thrombotic thrombocytopenic purpura is rare in children. Treatment for ITP consists of observation and/or gamma globulin and steroids. Splenectomy is reserved for the most severe and chronic forms.

395. The answer is a. *(Behrman, 16/e, pp. 981–983, 526–527, 1523. McMillan, 3/e, 367, 1475–1476, 1479–1480. Rudolph, 20/e pp. 768–772, 1192, 1243.)* Thrombocytopenia and hemolytic anemia are common manifestations of the TORCH (toxoplasmosis, rubella, cytomegalovirus, and herpes simplex) infections as well as congenital syphilis. Both increased platelet destruction and impaired production of platelets may be the mechanisms involved. Some mothers who have had ITP and who have high levels of antiplatelet antibody in the maternal plasma can give birth to thrombocytopenic infants because of transplacental crossing of antiplatelet IgG antibody. The syndrome of congenital amegakaryocytic thrombocytopenia and bilateral absence of the radii (TAR syndrome) is a well-known entity. Maternal ingestion of aspirin can lead to bleeding in the newborn, not as a result of thrombocytopenia but as a consequence of transient impairment of the infant's platelet aggregation. Neither chlamydial conjunctivitis nor nasolacrimal duct stenosis is usually associated with thrombocytopenia.

396. The answer is b. (*Behrman, 16/e, p. 1460. McMillan, 3/e, pp. 1447–1448, 1451–1453. Rudolph, 20/e, pp. 1209–1212.*) The concentration of hemoglobin A_2 is increased in β-thalassemia trait. In severe iron deficiency, hemoglobin A_2 may be decreased. In mild-to-moderate iron deficiency, the level of hemoglobin A_2 is normal. The level is also normal in sickle cell anemia, chronic systemic illness, and lead poisoning.

397. The answer is a. (*Behrman, 16/e, pp. 1520–1522. McMillan, 3/e, pp. 1477–1479, 1488, 1490–1491, 1493–1507, 2162–2165, 2176–2177, Rudolph, 20/e, pp. 486–489, 497, 1241–1242, 1271–1275.*) The mean age of presentation of ITP is 6 years. Patients look well except for petechial rash. Patients with acute lymphoblastic leukemia frequently have symptoms of pallor and fever in addition to bleeding. Nearly 50 percent of them have hepatomegaly and splenomegaly. CBC reveals anemia, leukocytosis or leukopenia, and thrombocytopenia. DIC is secondary to a severe underlying disease, such as fulminant bacterial sepsis with hypotension or profound hypoxia. Patients invariably appear ill and have leukocytosis, thrombocytopenia, and abnormal coagulation studies (e.g., prolonged PT and PTT, decreased fibrinogen concentration, and elevated fibrin split products) Patients with Henoch-Schönlein purpura have symptoms of skin rash and abdominal or joint pain. The rash is usually urticarial and purpuric and present over the buttocks or lower extremities. The platelet count is normal or elevated. SLE is very rare in a 3-year-old child. Findings include fever, joint pain, and skin rash. CBC can reveal anemia, leukopenia, and thrombocytopenia.

398. The answer is e. (*Behrman, 16/e, pp. 1489–1491. McMillan, 3/e, pp. 1455–1456, 2086. Rudolph, 20/e, pp. 1216–1217.*) Synthesis of the red cell enzyme glucose-6-phosphate dehydrogenase (G6PD) is determined by genes on the X chromosome, and the pattern of inheritance is X-linked recessive. The enzyme found in most populations is termed G6PDB+. There are over 380 deficient variants of the enzyme affecting over 100 million people worldwide, among them: G6PDA+, a mutant enzyme affecting about 13 percent of African-American males and 2 percent of African-American females; G6PDB or Mediterranean, a deficient mutant occurring among Middle Eastern, African, and Asian groups; and G6PD Canton occurring in 5 percent of Chinese.

In people with G6PDB+, enzyme activity is reduced to 50 percent during the 120-day life span of the erythrocyte. In persons affected with all G6PD deficiency variants, enzyme activity is always 10 percent of normal or less. Deficiency of G6PD compromises the generation of reduced glutathione, and upon exposure to oxidant agents such as sulfa drugs, antimalarials, nitrofurans, naphthalene mothballs, or infection, a hemolytic episode usually occurs. The degree of hemolysis depends on the nature of the oxidant and severity of the enzyme deficiency. In African-Americans, the older, more G6PD-deficient cells are destroyed, but since young cells have sufficient enzyme to prevent further red cell destruction even if the inciting factor is still present, the hemolytic crisis is usually self-limited. Blood transfusion may be unnecessary.

In African-Americans, premature testing for the enzyme immediately after a hemolytic episode can lead to a false negative result since the newly produced red cells in the circulation have a higher G6PD enzyme activity. The older red cells containing Heinz bodies (insoluble precipitates resulting from oxidation), the "bite cells" (red cells after the removal of the Heinz bodies), and cell fragments are removed from the circulation within 3 to 4 days. In the severe Mediterranean type, young as well as old red cells are enzyme-deficient. Recovery is signaled by the appearance of reticulocytes and a rise in hemoglobin.

399. The answer is d. (*Behrman, 16/e, pp. 1479–1483. McMillan, 3/e, pp. 1450–1451. Rudolph, 20/e, pp. 1203–1207.*) Acute splenic sequestration is a serious complication of sickle cell disease, usually occurring in patients under 5 years of age. Sudden massive pooling of blood in the splenic vasculature leads to hypovolemia and circulatory collapse. Early detection of splenomegaly by parents who have been taught the technique of abdominal palpation is an important aspect of patient management. The ability of the spleen to opsonize and phagocytize encapsulated organisms, particularly *Streptococcus pneumoniae* and *Haemophilus influenzae* b, is impaired in children with sickle cell disease as early as 6 months of age, and as a result, they are at an increased risk of infection with these organisms. A temperature of

38.5°C to 39°C (101.3°F to 102.2°F) calls for emergency evaluation even if the child does not look very sick. Without treatment, death from overwhelming sepsis, commonly due to pneumococcus, can occur within hours. Prophylactic oral penicillin early in infancy has been used to prevent pneumococcal infection. Polyvalent pneumococcal vaccine is started at the age of 2 years. Unfortunately, unconjugated polysaccharide vaccines are not good immunogens in infancy and early childhood, an especially critical period for patients with poor splenic function. Invasive *Haemophilus influenzae* b infections have been responsible for significant morbidity and mortality in patients with sickle cell disease. Special efforts should be made to immunize these children, as well as other immunocompromised children, with Hib vaccine as soon as they enter the health care system, even if they are over 5 years of age. Folic acid requirement is increased in sickle cell disease (as in all hemolytic anemias) and, therefore, supplementation is prudent. Vitamin B_{12} supplementation is not necessary, tetracycline is contraindicated because of damage to teeth; meningococcal vaccine is not indicated in children less than 2 years of age; and immunoglobulins have no place in the therapy of this condition.

400. The answer is a. *(Behrman, 16/e, pp. 519–521. McMillan, 3/e, pp. 359–362. Rudolph, 20/e, pp. 1168–1170, 1176–1180, 1203–1207.)* The absence of a major blood group incompatibility and the finding of a normal reticulocyte count argue strongly in favor of a recent fetomaternal transfusion, probably at the time of delivery. A Betke-Kleihauer stain for fetal hemoglobin-containing red cells in the mother's blood would confirm the diagnosis. After birth, erythropoiesis ceases, and the progressive decline in hemoglobin values, reaching a nadir at 6 to 8 weeks of age, has been termed physiologic anemia of infancy. Iron-deficiency anemia is common in the term infant between 9 and 24 months of age when the iron stores derived from circulating hemoglobin have been exhausted and an exogenous dietary source of iron has not been provided. The manifestations of sickle cell disease do not appear until 4 to 6 months of life, coincident with the replacement of fetal hemoglobin with sickle hemoglobin.

401. The answer is a. *(Behrman, 16/e, pp. 1543–1548. McMillan, 3/e, pp. 1493–1507. Rudolph, 20/e, pp. 1269–1271.)* Age less than 12 months or more than 10 to 15 years, the presence at diagnosis of central nervous system leukemia or a white blood cell count of 100,000/mm³ or higher, and the appearance of a mediastinal mass all indicate a poor prognosis for children who have acute lymphocytic leukemia. The first two prognostic factors listed above are the most reliable. Hyperdiploidy with more than 50 chromosomes is a good prognostic factor for treatment with antimetabolic-based chemotherapy. Most of the children with these poor prognostic signs have the thymic (T cell) variety of the disease. In addition to the conventionally employed regimen of prednisone and vincristine, other chemotherapeutic agents should be administered. A smaller fraction of these patients with poor prognostic features can be expected to achieve long-term disease-free survival, and once they relapse, many fail to go into remission despite aggressive chemotherapy. Bone marrow transplantation offers hope in some cases.

402. The answer is b. *(Behrman, 16/e, pp. 1554–1556. McMillan, 3/e, pp. 1515–1517. Rudolph, 20/e, pp. 1284–1286.)* An abdominal mass is palpated in 85 percent of patients with Wilms' tumor; abdominal pain is present in 40 percent, hypertension in about 60 percent, and hematuria in 12 percent to 24 percent. Because of the association of hemihypertrophy and aniridia with Wilms' tumor, children with these findings should be followed with periodic physical examinations and abdominal sonograms, especially during their first 5 years. Wilms' tumor and aniridia are associated with abnormalities in chromosome 11. Neuroblastoma should also be considered in the differential diagnosis of abdominal mass, especially if fever, irritability, bone pain, limp, and diarrhea are present.

403. The answer is d. *(Behrman, 16/e, pp. 1519–1520. McMillan, 3/e, p. 1488. Rudolph, 20/e, p. 1251.)* The clinical history and blood-smear findings (fragmented cells and few platelets) presented in the question are typical of disseminated intravascular coagulation. The disorder, which can be triggered by endotoxin shock, results ultimately in the initiation of the intrinsic clotting mechanism and the generation of thrombin (prolonged PT and PTT, decreased fibrinogen concentration, and an increase in fibrin split products). Fibrin deposited in the microcirculatory system can lead to tissue ischemia and necrosis, further capillary damage, release of thromboplastic substances, and increased thrombin generation. Simultaneous activation of the fibrinolytic system produces increased amounts of fibrin split products, which inhibit thrombin activity. Of utmost importance in the treatment of children who have disseminated intravascular coagulation is the management of the condition that precipitated the disorder.

404. The answer is d. *(Behrman, 16/8, pp. 614–615, 651–652, 666. McMillan, 3/e, pp. 1464–1465. Rudolph, 20/e, p. 1232.)* Some common causes of eosinophilia in the peripheral blood smear include asthma, recurrent urticaria, infantile eczema, serum sickness, angioneurotic edema, helminth infections, collagen vascular disease, and some neoplasms. Allergic rhinitis can cause eosinophilia in nasal secretions, but usually does not cause peripheral eosinophilia.

405. The answer is b. *(Behrman, 16/e, pp. 513–517, 1475–1477, 1479–1483, 1488. McMillan, 3/e, pp. 1450–1451, 1453–1455. Rudolph, 20/e, pp. 1203–1207, 1213–1214, 1219.)* Spherocytosis can be seen in hyperthermia, hereditary spherocytosis, G6PD deficiency, or ABO incompatibility. Hyperbilirubinemia has been associated with black preterm infants with G6PD deficiency. The blood smear of the affected infant usually reveals nucleated red cells, spherocytes, poikilocytes, "blister" cells, and fragmented cells. Neonatal hyperbilirubinemia occurs in about 50 percent of patients with hereditary spherocytosis. Spherocytosis occurs in ABO incompatibility but not in Rh incompatibility. The hemolytic manifestations of ABO incompatibility and hereditary spherocytosis are very similar. The blood types of the mother and of the infant should be determined along with the results of a direct Coombs' test on the infant and the presence or absence of a family history of hemolytic disease (spherocytosis). Sickle cell disease would not be expected to cause problems in newborns due to protection by fetal hemoglobin.

406. The answer is a. *(Behrman, 16/e, pp. 1469–1471. McMillan, 3/e, p. 1447–1448. Rudolph, 20/e, pp. 1176–1180.)* Iron-deficiency anemia is the most common nutritional deficiency in children between 9 and 15 months of age. Low availability of dietary iron, impaired absorption of iron related to frequent infections, high requirements for iron for growth, and, occasionally, blood losses, all favor the development of iron deficiency in infants. A history regarding anemia in the family, blood loss, and gestational age and weight can help to establish the cause of an anemia. The strong likelihood is that anemia in a 1-year-old child is nutritional in origin, and its cause will be suggested by a detailed nutritional history.

407. The answer is b. (*Behrman, 16/e, pp. 1469–1471. McMillan, 3/e, p. 1447–1448. Rudolph, 20/e, pp. 1176–1180.*) Response to a therapeutic trial of iron is an appropriate and cost-effective method of diagnosing iron-deficiency anemia. A prompt reticulocytosis and rise in hemoglobin and hematocrit follow the administration of an oral preparation of ferrous sulfate. Intramuscular iron dextran should be reserved for situations in which compliance cannot be achieved. This is because this treatment is expensive, painful, and no more effective than oral iron. Dietary modifications, such as limiting the intake of cow's milk and including iron-fortified cereals along with a mixed diet, are appropriate long-term measures, but they will not make enough iron available to replenish iron stores. The gradual onset of iron-deficiency anemia enables a child to adapt to surprisingly low hemoglobin concentrations. Transfusion is rarely indicated unless a child becomes symptomatic or is further compromised by a superimposed infection. When the iron available for production of hemoglobin is limited, free protoporphyrins accumulate in the blood. Levels of erythrocyte protoporphyrin (EP) are also elevated in lead poisoning. Iron-deficiency anemia can be differentiated from lead intoxication by measuring blood lead, which should be less than 10 μg/dL.

408. The answer is c. (*Behrman, 16/e, pp. 1519–1520. McMillan, 3/e, p. 1448. Rudolph, 20/e, pp. 1241–1242, 1245–1249, 1251.*) The prolongation of PT, aPTT, and TT excludes the diagnosis of ITP. PT tests principally for factors I, II, V, VII, and X and is not prolonged in hemophilia A (factor VIII deficiency) or hemophilia B (factor IX deficiency). In vitamin K deficiency, there is a decrease in the production of factors II, VII, IX, and X, and PT and aPTT are prolonged. The thrombin time, which tests for conversion of fibrinogen to fibrin, however, should be normal and the platelet count should also be normal. In DIC, there is consumption of fibrinogen; factors II, V, and VIII; and platelets. Therefore, there is prolongation of PT, aPTT, and TT and a decrease in factor VIII level and platelet count. In addition, the titer of fibrin split production is usually increased.

409. The answer is c. (*Behrman, 16/e, p. 1538. Rudolph, 20/e, p. 1267.*) The main toxicities of vincristine include peripheral neuropathy, constipation, jaw pain, and inappropriate antidiuretic hormone secretion. The major side effects of prednisone include cushingoid facies, truncal obesity, salt and water retention, hypertension, increased susceptibility to infection, gastric irritation, and osteoporosis. The toxicity of methotrexate is dependent on the dose, schedule, and route of administration. The major toxicities include gastrointestinal mucositis, bone marrow suppression, skin erythema, and hepatic dysfunction. 6-Mercaptopurine can cause nausea, vomiting, marrow suppression, and hepatic dysfunction. Doxorubicin (Adriamycin) can lead to alopecia, nausea, vomiting, stomatitis, tissue necrosis (if drug extravasates), and bone marrow suppression. The dose-limiting factor is cardiotoxicity, and the risk of cardiotoxicity increases at cumulative doses of doxorubicin above 550 mg/m^2.

410. The answer is d. *(Behrman, 16/e, pp. 1548–1550. McMillan, 3/e, pp. 1464–1465, 1507–1509. Rudolph, 20/e, pp. 1232, 1281–1284.)* In underdeveloped countries, the peak incidence of Hodgkin's disease is under 10 years of age; however, in the developed countries, the peak incidence occurs in late adolescence and young adulthood. Blood counts are usually normal, but eosinophilia can occur. Systemic symptoms of Hodgkin's disease include fever, night sweats, malaise, weight loss, and pruritus. In the Ann Arbor staging system, however, only fever, night sweats, and weight loss are considered significant systemic symptoms that have prognostic importance. In most instances, the initial mode of spread of Hodgkin's disease is predictable involvement of contiguous lymphoid tissue. The objective of surgical staging is to determine whether there is occult intraabdominal disease in patients who clinically have only apparent supradiaphragmatic involvement. The information provided by staging laparotomy is important if radiation therapy is the only modality of treatment contemplated. In patients who have obvious intraabdominal disease by noninvasive studies (such as CT scan or lymphangiogram) or obvious metastases outside the lymphatic system (e.g., bone marrow), combination chemotherapy with or without radiation therapy is generally recommended and staging laparotomy is then not required.

411. The answer is c. *(Behrman, 16/3, pp. 1467–1468. McMillan, 3/e, pp. 1448–1449. Rudolph, 20/e, pp. 1181–1182.)* The finding of hypersegmented neutrophils in the peripheral blood is one of the most useful laboratory aids in making an early diagnosis of folate deficiency. Serum folate levels become low in weeks with an inadequate dietary source. The Pelger-Huët anomaly is an inherited disorder in which neutrophils have no more than two lobes. Neutrophils in severe bacterial infections have toxic granulation, Döhle's inclusion bodies, and cytoplasmic vacuoles. Methotrexate, phenytoin, trimethoprim, and birth control pills can be associated with megaloblastic anemia, but these patients are usually not healthy and an appropriate history will give diagnostic clues.

412–415. The answers are 412–c, 413–d, 414–a, 415–b. *(Behrman, 16/3, p. 1475–1477, 1479–1487, 1526–1527. McMillan, 3/e, pp. 1451–1454, 1466, 1468, 2091. Rudolph, 20/e, pp. 1172–1176, 1205, 1209–1214, 1233–1234.)* Howell-Jolly bodies (slide **C**) are small, spherical nuclear remnants seen in the reticulocytes and, rarely, erythrocytes of persons who have no spleen (due to congenital asplenia or splenectomy) or who have a poorly functioning spleen (e.g., in hyposplenism associated with sickle cell disease). Ultrafiltration of blood is a unique function of the spleen that cannot be assumed by other reticuloendothelial organs.

A target cell is an erythrocyte with a membrane that is too large for its hemoglobin content; a thin rim of hemoglobin at the cell's periphery and a small disk in the center give the cell a target-like appearance. Target cells, which are more resistant to osmotic fragility than are other erythrocytes, are seen in children who have β-thalassemia, hemoglobin C disease, or liver disease (e.g., obstructive jaundice or cirrhosis). Thalassemia major (slide **D**) can be diagnosed by the presence of poorly hemoglobinized normoblasts in addition to target cells in the peripheral blood.

Uniformly small microspherocyte (less than 6 μm in diameter) are typical of hereditary spherocytosis (slide **A**). Because of a decreased surface-to-volume ratio, these osmotically fragile red blood cells have an increased density of hemoglobin. Although spherical red blood cells also can appear in other hemolytic states (e.g., immune hemolytic anemia, microangiography, ABO incompatibility, and hypersplenism), their cellular volume is only irregularly augmented.

Although hemoglobin C disease (slide **B**) is frequently a mild disorder, target cells constitute a far greater percentage of total red blood cells than in thalassemia major.

ENDOCRINE, METABOLIC, AND GENETIC DISORDERS

Questions

DIRECTIONS: Each item below contains a question or incomplete statement followed by suggested responses. Select the **one best** response to each question.

416. Tyrosinosis, galactosemia, deficiency of alpha$_1$ antitrypsin, and fructosemia have as a primary feature common involvement of which organ of the body?

a.   skin
b.   lungs
c.   liver
d.   gonads
e.   hematologic system

417. A 12-year-old healthy Jewish girl is found on routine blood count to have a mild anemia, leukopenia, and thrombocytopenia. Physical examination reveals an enlarged spleen. An x-ray of the femur is described as a appearing to be an Erlenmeyer flask. Bone marrow examination shows abnormal cells. The diagnosis can be confirmed by measurement of activity of which of the following?

a.   sphingomyelinase activity
b.   hexosamidase A
c.   sulfatase A
d.   glucocerebrosidase
e.   ceramide trihexosidase

418. Which of the following statements about neonatal thyrotoxicosis is true?

a.   it occurs more commonly in girls than boys
b.   it is thought to be caused by cross-placental passage of maternal thyroid-stimulating immunoglobulins (TSI)
c.   it is often a life-long problem
d.   it is a mild condition and does not require specific therapy
e.   it does not occur when the mother is being treated with antithyroid drugs

419. True sexual precocity in girls is most likely to be caused by

a.   a feminizing ovarian tumor
b.   a gonadotropin-producing tumor
c.   a lesion of the central nervous system
d.   exogenous estrogens
e.   early onset of "normal" puberty (constitutional)

Items 420–421

420. The parents of a 14-year-old boy are concerned about his short stature and lack of sexual development. By history, you learn that his birth weight and length were 3 kg and 50 cm, respectively, and that he had a normal growth pattern, although he was always shorter than children his age. The physical examination is normal. His upper-to-lower segment ratio is 0.98. A small amount of fine axillary and pubic hair is present. There is no scrotal pigmentation; his testes measure 4.0 cm^3 and his penis is 6 cm in length. In this situation you should

a. measure pituitary gonadotropin
b. obtain CT scan of pituitary area
c. biopsy his testes
d. measure serum testosterone levels
e. reassure parents that the boy is normal

421. Which of the following is the most likely diagnosis for the patient in the previous question?

a. hypopituitarism
b. Klinefelter's syndrome
c. hypothyroidism
d. constitutionally short stature with delayed puberty
e. male Turner's syndrome

Items 422–423

422. A 13-year-old asymptomatic girl is found to have an enlarged thyroid. She states that the front of her neck has been growing slowly for more than a year. The most likely diagnosis is

a. iodine deficiency
b. congenital hypothyroidism
c. Graves' disease
d. exogenous ingestion of synthroid
e. lymphocytic (Hashimoto's) thyroiditis

423. Treatment for the patient in the previous question includes

a. iodine
b. synthroid if she becomes symptomatic
c. PTU (propylthiouracil)
d. psychiatry consult
e. surgical removal of thyroid

Items 424–425

424. A 10-year-old obese boy has central fat distribution, arrested growth, hypertension, plethora, purple striae, and osteoporosis. Which of the following disorders is most likely to be responsible for the clinical picture that this boy presents?

a. bilateral adrenal hyperplasia
b. adrenal adenoma
c. adrenal carcinoma
d. craniopharyngioma
e. ectopic adrenocorticotropin-producing tumor

425. Appropriate initial management of this young man is

a. measurement of evening cortisol levels
b. MRI of the adrenals
c. bilateral inferior petrosal blood sampling
d. MRI of the brain and pituitary
e. adrenal scintigraphy with radio-cholesterol

426. Which of the following is appropriate advice given to a couple with a 3-month-old child recently diagnosed by sweat chloride testing with cystic fibrosis?

a. have all siblings assessed for cystic fibrosis with sweat chloride testing
b. determine parental carrier state with DNA analysis for carrier state
c. determine siblings carrier state with DNA analysis
d. determine the couple's carrier state by sweat chloride testing
e. determine siblings' carrier state with sweat chloride testing

427. A 2-week-old female is noted to have a thin membrane adhering together the upper portion of labia minora. The most appropriate course of action for these labial adhesions is to

a. apply estrogen cream daily
b. refer for surgical repair
c. apply traction to the opposing labia until the adhesion breaks
d. evaluate the patient for congenital adrenal hyperplasia
e. do nothing as the lesions are of no consequence

428. Which of the following disorders of growth is characterized by a normal body proportion?

a. achondroplasia
b. Morquio's disease
c. hypothyroidism
d. growth hormone deficiency
e. Marfan's syndrome

429. Concerning human leukocyte antigen (HLA) compatibility in bone marrow transplant (BMT), which of the following statements is true?

a. there is a 1 in 2 chance that two siblings are HLA-matched
b. each parent is diploidentical to the child
c. identical twins are not necessarily HLA-matched
d. unrelated donors can occasionally be matched
e. it is always better to use a family member as a donor

430. A 13-year-old boy is below the 3rd percentile for height (50th percentile for age 9). Which of the following would give him the best prognosis for normal adult height?

a. a bone age of 9 years
b. a bone age of 13 years
c. a bone age of 15 years
d. being at the 50th percentile for weight
e. being at the 3rd percentile for weight

431. A 12-year-old girl has a mass in her neck. Physical examination reveals a thyroid nodule, but the rest of the gland is not palpable. A technetium scan reveals a "cold" nodule. The child appears to be euthyroid. Which of the following diagnoses is the LEAST likely?

a. simple adenoma
b. follicular carcinoma
c. papillary carcinoma
d. a cyst
e. dysgenetic thyroid gland

432. The child pictured has

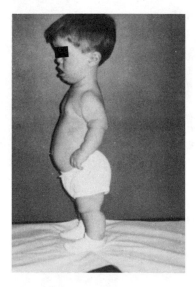

a. achondrogenesis
b. achondroplasia
c. metatrophic dwarfism
d. thanatophoric dwarfism
e. chondroectodermal dysplasia

433. A 6-month-old male infant with leukokoria and onset of strabismus is brought to the United States from a developing country. The family history reveals that his father had an eye and a leg removed. The most likely diagnosis is

a. coloboma of the choroid
b. retinal detachment
c. nematode endophthalmitis
d. retinoblastoma
e. persistent hyperplastic primary vitreous

434. Bone age will be advanced in short stature caused by which of the following?

a. environmental deprivation syndrome
b. hypopituitarism
c. hypothyroidism
d. congenital adrenal hyperplasia
e. chronic administration of glucocorticoids in high doses

435. Patients with pseudohypoparathyroidism are expected to have which of the following features?

a. hypercalcemia
b. hypophosphatemia
c. elevated concentrations of parathyroid hormone
d. advanced height age
e. rise in urinary phosphate excretion in response to the infusion of parathyroid hormone

436. A 15-year-old boy has been immobilized in a double hip spica for 6 weeks after having fractured his femur in a skiing accident. He has become depressed and listless during the past few days and has complained of nausea and constipation. He is found to have microscopic hematuria and a blood pressure of 150/100 mm Hg. You should

a. request a psychiatric evaluation
b. check blood pressure every 2 h for 2 days
c. collect urine for measurement of the calcium–creatinine ratio
d. order a renal sonogram and intravenous pyelogram (IVP)
e. measure 24 h urinary protein

437. Glycosylated hemoglobin (hemoglobin A_{1C}) is often used as an indicator of control in patients with diabetes mellitus. Its level usually reflects the blood concentration of glucose over the preceding

a. 8 h
b. 1 week
c. 1 month
d. 2 months
e. 6 months

Items 438–439

438. A 7-day-old boy is admitted to a hospital for evaluation of vomiting and dehydration. Physical examination is otherwise normal except for minimal hyperpigmentation of the nipples. Serum sodium and potassium concentrations are 120 mEq/L and 9 mEq/L, respectively; serum glucose is 120mg/dL. The most likely diagnosis is

a. pyloric stenosis
b. congenital adrenal hyperplasia
c. secondary hypothyroidism
d. panhypopituitarism
e. hyperaldosteronism

439. The diagnosis can be confirmed in this patient by

a. obtaining a barium swallow
b. measurement of 17-hydroxy-progesterone
c. measurement of T3, T4, and TSH
d. somatomedin C measurement
e. measurement of serum renin levels

440. An infant is brought to a hospital because her wet diapers turn black when they are exposed to air. Physical examination is normal. Urine is positive both for reducing substance and when tested with ferric chloride. This disorder is caused by a deficiency of

a. homogentisic acid oxidase
b. phenylalanine hydroxylase
c. l-histidine ammonia-lyase
d. ketoacid decarboxylase
e. isovaleryl-CoA dehydrogenase

441. Which of the following statements about Wilson's disease is true?

a. it is inherited as a sex-linked trait
b. in children, it usually presents with splenomegaly and overwhelming infection with encapsulated organisms
c. ceruloplasmin levels are typically increased
d. total serum copper concentration is usually high
e. it is often associated with renal disease (Fanconi's syndrome)

442. In which of the following phenotypic girls is body hair distribution typically normal?

a. congenital adrenal hyperplasia (adrenogenital syndrome)
b. Cushing's syndrome
c. androgen-producing ovarian tumor
d. testicular feminization — phenotypic female with intra-abdominal testes and 46,XY karyotype
e. administration of exogenous androgens

443. Which of the following laboratory findings is unusual in patients with simple (nutritional) rickets?

a. hypercalcemia
b. hyperphosphaturia
c. elevated levels of serum alkaline phosphatase
d. hypercalciuria
e. hypophosphatemia

444. Normal mentation is usually found with tall stature in which of the following syndromes listed below?

a. cerebral gigantism (Sotos' syndrome)
b. homocystinuria
c. XXY (Klinefelter's syndrome)
d. Marfan's syndrome
e. XYY

445. Neonatal hypoglycemia is common in premature infants and those small for gestational age. The most common cause of hypoglycemia in these infants is

a. inadequate stores of nutrients
b. adrenal immaturity
c. pituitary immaturity
d. insulin excess
e. glucagon deficiency

446. A 1-day-old infant develops tetany and convulsions. Serum calcium is 6.2 mg/dL. Which of the following diagnoses is the LEAST likely in this infant?

a. perinatal asphyxia
b. high phosphate intake
c. maternal diabetes mellitus
d. maternal hyperparathyroidism
e. prematurity

DIRECTIONS: Each group of questions below consists of lettered options followed by numbered items. For each numbered item, select the appropriate lettered option(s). Each lettered option may be used once, more than once, or not at all. **Choose exactly the number of options indicated following each item.**

Items 447–451

For each of the disorders listed below, select the serum concentration of calcium (Ca) and phosphate (PO_4) with which it is most likely to be associated.

a. low PO_4, normal Ca
b. low PO_4, high Ca
c. normal PO_4, low Ca
d. normal PO_4, normal Ca
e. high PO_4, low Ca

447. Vitamin D–resistant rickets
(SELECT 1 FINDING)

448. Pseudohypoparathyroidism
(SELECT 1 FINDING)

449. Osteogenesis imperfecta
(SELECT 1 FINDING)

450. Hyperparathyroidism
(SELECT 1 FINDING)

451. Medullary thyroid carcinoma with hypercalcitoninemia
(SELECT 1 FINDING)

Items 452–457

All the syndromes listed below are associated with obesity in children. For each of the other clinical findings that follow, select the syndrome with which it is most likely to be associated.

a. Prader-Willi syndrome
b. Laurence-Moon-Biedl syndrome
c. Cushing's syndrome
d. Fröhlich's syndrome
e. pseudohypoparathyroidism

452. Cataracts
(SELECT 1 SYNDROME)

453. Hypotonia
(SELECT 1 SYNDROME)

454. Polydactyly
(SELECT 1 SYNDROME)

455. Brachydactyly
(SELECT 1 SYNDROME)

456. Basal ganglia calcification
(SELECT 1 SYNDROME)

457. Retinitis pigmentosa
(SELECT 1 SYNDROME)

Items 458–463

For each of the following disorders, select the serum concentrations (mEq/L) of sodium (Na^+) and potassium (K^+) with which it is most likely to be associated in a dehydrated patient.

a. Na^+ 118, K^+ 7.5
b. Na^+ 125, K^+ 3.0
c. Na^+ 134, K^+ 6.0
d. Na^+ 144, K^+ 2.9
e. Na^+ 155, K^+ 5.5

458. Salt-losing 21-hydroxylase deficiency (adrenogenital syndrome)
(SELECT 1 FINDING)

459. Central diabetes insipidus
(SELECT 1 FINDING)

460. Nephrogenic diabetes insipidus
(SELECT 1 FINDING)

461. Hyperaldosteronism
(SELECT 1 FINDING)

462. Addison's disease (in crisis)
(SELECT 1 FINDING)

463. Glucose-6-phosphatase deficiency (von Gierke's disease)
(SELECT 1 FINDING)

Items 464–468

For each diagnosis that follows, select the mode of inheritance with which it is usually associated.

a. autosomal dominant
b. autosomal recessive
c. X-linked dominant
d. X-linked recessive
e. none of the above

464. Hypophosphatemic rickets
(SELECT 1 MODE)

465. Childhood polycystic kidneys and liver
(SELECT 1 MODE)

466. Systemic lupus erythematosus
(SELECT 1 MODE)

467. Cystinosis
(SELECT 1 MODE)

468. Adult-type polycystic kidneys
(SELECT 1 MODE)

Items 469–470

New discoveries made possible by advances in molecular genetics have broadened our understanding of nontraditional inheritance. Match the disease with the appropriate genetic mechanism below.

a. mitochondrial inheritance
b. mosaicism
c. genomic imprinting
d. sex chromosome imbalance

469. Myoclonic epilepsy with ragged red fibers
(SELECT 1 MECHANISM)

470. Prader-Willi and Angelman syndromes
(SELECT 1 MECHANISM)

Items 471–472

Select the first sign of pubertal changes in boys and girls.

a. enlargement of the testes
b. development of pubic hair
c. acne
d. development of breast buds
e. penile enlargement
f. ovulation
g. thickening of the vaginal mucosa
h. growth spurt

471. The first sign of pubertal development in a boy
SELECT 1 SIGN)

472. The first sign of pubertal development in a girl
(SELECT 1 SIGN)

Items 473–474

Match each patient with the appropriate findings.

a. tracheoesophageal fistula
b. endocardial cushion defect
c. short stature
d. lactose intolerance
e. increased incidence in younger mothers
f. a history of duodenal atresia at birth
g. heterochromia
h. panhypopituitarism
i. streak gonads
j. renal failure
k. increased incidence of cystic fibrosis
l. coarctation of the aorta

473. A child with Down syndrome
(SELECT 3 FINDINGS)

474. A child with Turner's syndrome
(SELECT 3 FINDINGS)

ENDOCRINE, METABOLIC, AND GENETIC DISORDERS

Answers

416. The answer is c. *(Behrman, 16/3, pp. 344–8, 407, 413–414. McMillan, 3/e, pp. 1198, 1210, 1747–1750, 1830–1831, 1859. Rudolph, 20/e, pp. 306–310, 1142–1144.)* Galactosemia, fructosemia, and tyrosinosis represent diseases in which a congenital deficiency of enzyme causes an interruption of a normal metabolic pathway and an accumulation of metabolic precursors that damage vital organs. The mode of inheritance of these disorders is autosomal recessive. In galactosemia and fructosemia, errors in carbohydrate metabolism cause the accumulation of toxic metabolites when specific dietary sugars are introduced (lactose in galactosemia; fructose and sucrose in fructosemia). Exclusion of the offending carbohydrate from the diet will prevent liver damage. In tyrosinemia type I, or tyrosinosis, the accumulation of tyrosine and its metabolites is associated with severe involvement of liver, kidney, and central nervous system. Manifestations of acute liver failure can appear in infancy. A chronic form of the disorder presents as progressive cirrhosis and leads to liver failure or hepatoma. Dietary management does not prevent liver disease. The course of liver disease when it does occur in deficiency of alpha1 antitrypsin is variable.

417. The answer is d. *(Behrman, 16/e, pp. 400–404. McMillan, 3/e, pp. 1876–1877. Rudolph, 20/e, pp. 336–337, 341.)* Gaucher's disease is characterized by β glucocerebrosidase deficiency, which causes an abnormal accumulation of glucocerebroside in the reticuloendothelial system. Bone marrow aspirate shows the typical Gaucher cells engorged with glucocerebroside. Replacement of marrow leads to anemia, leukopenia, and thrombocytopenia. The liver and spleen can also be involved. Serum acid phosphatase is elevated. X-ray demonstrates an Erlenmeyer flask appearance of the long bones. The diagnosis of Gaucher's disease is confirmed by the absence of glucocerebrosidase activity in leukocytes, in cultured skin fibroblasts, and in liver cells. Prenatal diagnosis by enzyme analysis is now possible. In the most common form of Gaucher's disease, adult type I, there is no involvement of the central nervous system. Therefore, MRI of the brain is not indicated. Sphingomyelinase deficiency causes type A Niemann-Pick disease; hexosaminidase A deficiency causes Sandhoff's disease; sulfatase A deficiency causes juvenile metachromatic leukodystrophy; and serum trihexosidase causes Fabry's disease.

418. The answer is b. *(Behrman, 16/e, pp. 1711–1712, McMillan, 3/e, pp. 355, 1809. Rudolph, 20/e, p. 1769.)* Infants born to thyrotoxic mothers can be hypothyroid, euthyroid, or hyperthyroid. Neonatal thyrotoxicosis usually disappears within 2 to 4 months as the concentration of thyroid-stimulating immunoglobulins (7S gammaglobulin) diminishes. Unlike TSI, thyroid-stimulating hormone (TSH) does not cross the placenta. All forms of thyrotoxicosis are more common in females with the exception of neonatal thyrotoxicosis, which has an equal sex distribution. In severely affected infants, the disease could be fatal if not treated vigorously and promptly.

419. The answer is e. *(Behrman, 16/e, pp. 1687–1690. McMillan, 3/e, pp. 1772–1774. Rudolph, 20/e, pp. 1795–1799.)* The term true sexual precocity implies that gonads have matured in response to the secretion of pituitary gonadotropins and have begun secreting sex steroids, causing the development of secondary sexual characteristics. Thus, ovarian tumors and exogenous estrogens, which suppress the function of the pituitary gland, do not cause true precocious puberty. In girls, the most common form of true precocious puberty is idiopathic and is thought to be caused by early maturation of an otherwise normal hypothalamic–pituitary–gonadal feedback system. In boys, true precocious puberty is relatively rare and is more likely to be caused by lesions of the central nervous system. Gonadotropin-producing tumors, which are very rare, can cause true precocious puberty in both sexes.

420. The answer is e. *(Behrman, 16/e, p. 1679. McMillan, 3/e, pp. 1775–1780. Rudolph, 20/e, pp. 1800–1802.)* A record of the sequential pattern of growth in height is very helpful in the differential diagnosis of a child with short stature. A child with constitutionally short stature and delayed puberty will have a consistent rate of growth below but parallel to the average for his or her age, whereas patients with organic disease do not follow a given percentile but progressively deviate from their prior growth percentile. A knowledge of the patterns of growth and sexual maturation of family members is helpful because such patterns are often familial. Puberty is said to be delayed in males if physical changes are not apparent by 14 years of age. Identification of the earliest signs of sexual maturation by means of careful physical examination avoids unnecessary workup. In this case, measurement of pituitary gonadotropins is unnecessary because the child already shows evidence of pubertal development (a testicular length of more than 2.5 cm, volume 3.0 cm^3). The single most useful laboratory test is the determination of bone age. In constitutionally short stature with delayed pubertal maturation, the bone age is equal to the height age, both of which are behind chronologic age. In familial short stature, bone age is greater than height age and equal to chronologic age. In a child at any age, the administration of human chorionic gonadotropin (hCG) will stimulate interstitial cells of testes to produce testosterone, thereby serving as a method of assessing testicular function. The finding of testicular enlargement is evidence of pituitary secretion of gonadotropins and of testicular responsiveness and obviates the need for administration of hCG. Elevated serum gonadotropins are found in children 12 years of age or older who have primary hypogonadism (Klinefelter's syndrome, bilateral gonadal failure from trauma or infection). Because the secretion of gonadotropins is not constant but occurs in spurts, children with constitutional delay of puberty may have normal or low levels of gonadotropins.

421. The answer is d. *(Behrman, 16/e, pp. 1675–1680, 1703–1704, 1747–1748. McMillan, 3/e, pp. 1775, 1779, 1808–1809, 2231, 2243. Rudolph, 20/e, pp. 1683–1687, 1764–1765, 1785–1786, 1800–1802.)* In Klinefelter's syndrome, the testes are smaller than normal for age and feel firm and fibrotic. Physical examination often reveals a eunuchoid body habitus and reduced upper-to-lower body segment ratio secondary to a long lower segment. Diagnosis is established by means of buccal smear and karyotyping. Levels of luteinizing hormone are elevated after 12 years of age. Hypothyroidism and hypopituitarism are associated with a deviation from the previously established growth pattern in addition to delayed bone age and other abnormal findings on physical examination. In the so-called male Turner's syndrome, many of the features of classic Turner's syndrome, which occurs in females, are present. In addition, the testes are hypoplastic and often undescended. A consistent growth pattern and normal upper-to-lower body segment ratio support the diagnosis of constitutionally short stature. Bone age consistent with height age rather than chronologic age is also a supportive finding. Reassurance that normal sexual development will occur and that a normal adult height (usually a mid parental height) will be attained is frequently the only therapy indicated.

422–423. The answers are 422–e, 423–b. *(Behrman, 16/e, pp. 1704–1705. McMillan, 3/e, pp. 1808–1809. Rudolph, 20/e, pp. 1762–1763.)* Lymphocytic thyroiditis is a typical organ-specific autoimmune disease characterized by lymphocytic infiltration of the thyroid gland, with or without goiter. It is the most common cause of juvenile hypothyroidism, peaking in adolescence, and affecting as many as 1 percent of school children. The condition is 4 to 7 times more prevalent in girls than in boys and may persist for many years without symptoms. Patients are initially euthyroid but with the eventual atrophy of the gland, they become hypothyroid. Spontaneous remission can occur in one third of the affected adolescents. Hashimoto's thyroiditis is not related to endemic goiter caused by iodine deficiency.

Autoimmune thyroiditis is associated with many other autoimmune disorders; its association with Addison's disease and insulin-dependent diabetes mellitus is called type II polyglandular autoimmune disease (Schmidt's syndrome). Family clusters of autoimmune thyroiditis are common; nearly 50 percent of the patients have siblings with antithyroid antibodies.

In Hashimoto's thyroiditis, thyroid function tests are often normal, although an elevated TSH level may be seen in a euthyroid child. With progressive thyroid failure, T_3 and T_4 levels drop and the TSH level rises. Most patients have titers of thyroid antimicrosomal antibodies; elevated antithyroglobulin titers occur infrequently. Blocking TSH antibodies are thought to be related to development of hypothyroidism. Congenital rubella infection can cause late-onset thyroiditis and hypothyroidism on an autoimmune basis. Antirubella antibodies cannot be used for diagnostic purposes in this 13-year-old child because she has probably been immunized with the attenuated vaccine or may have had rubella in childhood.

424–425. The answers are 424–a, 425–a. *(Behrman, 16/e, pp. 1737–1739. McMillan, 3/e, pp. 1819–1820. Rudolph, 20/e, pp. 1731–1734.)* Although the administration of exogenous adrenocorticotropic hormone or of glucocorticoids is the most common cause of Cushing's syndrome, it can also be caused by bilateral adrenal hyperplasia. In the latter case, the concentration of adrenocorticotropic hormone can be normal or high. The basic abnormality, however, is thought to be in the hypothalamic–pituitary axis, not the adrenal gland, because a distinct pituitary adenoma is found in some patients. Furthermore, many patients who have undergone bilateral adrenalectomy develop Nelson's syndrome (invasive pituitary adenoma) despite receiving adequate cortisol replacement. If the patient were an infant, however, the most likely answer would have been an adrenal carcinoma.

The initial management of this child would be to measure evening cortisol levels which, in a normal child, are expected to be less than 50 percent of the 8:00 AM value. Additionally, 24-hour excretion of 17-hydroxy-corticosteroids is almost always increased. In difficult-to-diagnose cases, a dexamethasone suppression test can be required. After the diagnosis has been established, further testing is indicated to determine if the condition is ACTH-dependent or ACTH-independent. At that point, corticotropin-releasing hormone testing and imaging will be required.

426. The answer is c. *(Behrman, 16/e, pp. 1315–1327. McMillan, 3/e, pp. 1242–1254. Rudolph, 20/e, pp. 1640–1650.)* Cystic fibrosis (CF) has an autosomal recessive pattern of inheritance; both parents are usually heterozygous and the affected child may be a homozygote (two copies of the same mutation) or a compound heterozygote (one copy of each of two different mutations). The ΔF508 mutation, present in about 70 percent of North American whites, is the most common. In Europe, the incidence of this mutation ranges from 40 percent to 80 percent in different population groups. There are many other mutations that vary in specific ethnic groups.

Identification of a CF mutation in both chromosomes, whether homozygous or compound heterozygous, would be diagnostic in 72 percent. DNA testing can help predict manifestations of the disease, especially pancreatic involvement. Pancreatic insufficiency is present in 99 percent of patients who are homozygous for DF508, in 72 percent who are compound homozygous for DF508, and only in 32 percent who do not carry the DF508 mutation. DNA analysis for carrier testing is now recommended for relatives of CF patients and for reproductive partners of carriers. Its role in mass population screening is controversial. The sweat test is diagnostic in virtually all cases of classic CF and is equally useful in all ethnic groups, but it is not useful in detecting heterozygotes. DNA testing is of value for postmortem investigations as well as in sick premature infants and other patients when sweat collection is unsuccessful.

427. The answer is a. *(Behrman, 16/e, pp. 1660–1661.)* This common condition is diagnosed when a central line of adherence is noted from the area inferior to the clitoris to the fourchette. It is a common, asymptomatic condition seen in girls less than 6 years of age. Labial adhesions can be responsible for vulvovaginitis and increased urinary tract infections in girls because pooling of urine in the vagina. Treatment with topical estrogen cream daily results in resolution of this problem. Mechanical separation is not advisable under normal circumstances.

428. The answer is d. *(Behrman, 16/e, pp. 421–422, 1675–1678, 1698–1704, 2121–2123, 2131–2132. McMillan, 3/e, pp. 1782–1783, 1790–1791, 1808–1809, 1873, 1893–1895, 2142. Rudolph, 20/e, pp. 360–361, 377–381, 392–394, 1697, 1764–1765.)* Alteration of body proportion results from selective regional rates of growth at different stages during the developmental period. At birth, the head is large for the body size, the limbs are short, and the upper-to-lower segment ratio (crown to pubis/pubis to heel) of 1.7 is high. As the growth of the limbs exceeds that of the trunk from infancy to adolescence, there is a change in body proportions reflected in the upper-to-lower segment ratios: 1.3 at 3 years, 1.1 at 6 years, and 1.0 at 10 years of age. In achondroplasia, there is a disproportion between the limbs and the trunk; that is, the limbs are relatively short. The head in this condition is also disproportionately large. Achondroplasia is the most common genetic skeletal dysplasia. This disorder has an autosomal dominant mode of inheritance. Marfan's syndrome is a serious disease of connective tissue that is inherited in the autosomal dominant mode. The predominant findings in this condition are bilateral subluxation of the lens, dilatation of the aortic root, and disproportionately long limbs in comparison with the trunk. The decreased upper-to-lower segment ratio in Marfan's syndrome reflects this relative increase in the length of the legs as compared with the trunk. Morquio's syndrome is one of the mucopolysaccharidoses. Abnormal amounts of keratan sulfate accumulate as a result of an enzyme deficiency, and widespread storage of this material in the body results in problems in morphogenesis and function. Skeletal malformations are similar to those seen in osteochondrodysplasias, namely, short trunk with short stature, marked slowing of growth, severe scoliosis, pectus carinatum, and short neck. Thyroid hormone is necessary for physical growth and development and, along with sex hormones, has an essential role in development of bone and linear growth. Thyroid deficiency results in delayed puberty in most cases and in stunting of growth with persistence of immature body proportions. In growth hormone deficiency, the upper-to-lower segment ratio is normal.

429. The answer is d. *(Behrman, 16/e, pp. 634–644. McMillan, 3/e, pp. 1505–1507. Rudolph, 20/e, pp. 1261–1262.)* In bone marrow transplantation, human leukocyte antigen (HLA) compatibility is important in preventing graft rejection and graft-versus-host disease (GVHD). The marrow donor can be the patient (autologous transplant), an identical twin in which, by definition, HLA is identical (syngeneic transplant), or a histocompatible donor, usually a sibling (allogeneic transplant). The HLA complex, a series of genetic loci on the short arm of chromosome 6, is usually inherited as a group or haplotype in a codominant mendelian fashion, one from each parent. Statistically, then, 25 percent of siblings will inherit the same haplotype from each parent and, therefore, be HLA-matched and histocompatible. If the donor and recipient share only one haplotype, they are termed haploidentical, a situation that pertains to a parent–child pair, for example. Identification of potential donors has been facilitated by the International Bone Marrow Transplant Registry, a computerized list of the names and HLA types of tens of thousands of persons. In a highly HLA-disparate family, it can be preferable to look for a closely matched unrelated donor.

430. The answer is a. *(Behrman, 16/e, pp. 56, 59–60. McMillan, 3/e, pp. 1776–1780, 1790–1791. Rudolph, 20/e, p. 1696.)* The determination of bone age by the radiographic examination of ossification centers provides a measure of a child's level of growth that is independent of his or her chronologic age. Height age is the age that corresponds to the 50th percentile for a child's height. When bone age and height age are equally retarded several years behind chronologic age, a child is described as having constitutional short stature. Such a child is usually shorter than peers in adolescence because of the delayed growth spurt, but the prognosis for normal adult height is excellent because there is still the potential for growth. Detailed questioning will usually identify other family members with a history of delayed growth and sexual maturation but with ultimately normal stature. Children with genetic or familial short stature grow at an adequate rate, but remain small throughout life; their ultimate height is consistent with predictions based on parental heights. Bone age is within the limits of normal for chronologic age, and puberty occurs at the normal time. In all cases, a thorough history and physical examination are necessary to identify any other cause of growth delay.

431. The answer is e. *(Behrman, 16/e, pp. 1698, 1712–1713. McMillan, 3/e, pp. 1806, 1811–1812. Rudolph, 20/e, pp. 1757, 1770–1772.)* A dysgenetic thyroid gland can appear as a neck mass; as a rule, however, it is functional and, thus, does not appear as a "cold" nodule on thyroid scan. A "cold" thyroid nodule can be a benign or malignant lesion. With the exception of anaplastic carcinomas, most thyroid malignancies are slow growing. The incidence of thyroid malignancy in children appears to be decreasing, possibly as a result of a decrease in the exposure of children to x-rays.

432. The answer is b. *(Behrman, 16/e, pp. 2121–2123. McMillan, 3/e, pp. 2141–2147. Rudolph, 20/e, pp. 381–382.)* Achondroplasia, occurring with an incidence of approximately 1 in every 26,000 live births, is the most common genetic form of skeletal dysplasia. Affected persons bear a striking resemblance to one another and are identified by their extremely short extremities; prominent foreheads; short, stubby fingers; and marked lumbar lordosis. Although they go through normal puberty, affected females must have children by cesarean section because of the pelvic deformity.

433. The answer is d. *(Behrman, 16/e, pp. 1561–1562. McMillan, 3/e, pp. 676–677, 1525–1527. Rudolph, 20/e, p. 2105.)* Although all the listed options can produce the symptoms described, the family history supports the diagnosis of retinoblastoma, the most common intraocular tumor in children. Early detection can result in a survival rate of over 75 percent. The pattern of inheritance of retinoblastoma is complicated: the hereditary form of the disease can be transmitted by means of autosomal dominant inheritance from an affected parent, or from an unaffected parent carrying the gene, or from a new germinal mutation. Familial occurrences are usually bilateral. A second primary tumor develops in 15 percent to 90 percent of survivors of bilateral retinoblastoma, the most common of which is osteosarcoma increasing with time. Retinoblastoma is associated with a mutation or deletion of the long arm of chromosome 13. In addition to specialized ophthalmologic care, management of retinoblastoma includes molecular genetic investigation of the family to identify those who have inherited the tumor-predisposing retinoblastoma gene.

434. The answer is d. (*Behrman, 16/e, pp. 59–60, 1675–1680, 1698–1704, 1729–1736, 1738. McMillan, 3/e, pp. 1776–1780. Rudolph, 20/e, pp. 1683–1687, 1725–1729, 1764–1765, 1792–1793.*) The appearance and union of the various centers of ossification follows a fairly definite pattern and time schedule from birth through adolescence. This process provides, through x-ray studies, a valuable criterion for estimating normal and abnormal growth. The skeletal maturity of any person is known as the bone age. Bone maturation is particularly influenced by the androgenic and estrogenic hormones. In congenital adrenal hyperplasia, a deficiency of enzyme (21-hydroxylase in 80 percent of cases) causes an interruption in the pathway for production of cortisol; the end result is hypersecretion of androgenic precursors and clinical manifestations of virilism and protein anabolism. In both males and females, muscles are well developed and there is rapid growth in stature with marked acceleration of osseous maturation. The result is early closure of epiphyses and failure to achieve full growth. Thyroid hormone appears to act as a primary stimulant to skeletal maturation. Deficiency of thyroxine results in marked retardation of bone age. Failure to thrive as a consequence of profound environmental deprivation is characterized by very low levels of circulating pituitary hormones and is associated with a delay in skeletal maturation. Removal of the child from the abnormal environment results in dramatic catch-up growth and a rapid return of hormone levels to normal. Glucocorticoid excess, either endogenous or exogenous, is associated with a decrease in the rate of growth and a delay in the onset of puberty. These effects appear to be mediated at end-organ sites as part of the catabolic effects of these steroids.

435. The answer is c. (*Behrman, 16/e, pp. 1718–1719. McMillan, 3/e, pp. 1620–1621. Rudolph, 20/e, p. 1842.*) Patients with pseudohypoparathyroidism have the chemical findings of hypoparathyroidism (low calcium, high phosphorus), but parathyroid hormone levels are high, indicating resistance to the action of this hormone. Thus, parathyroid hormone infusion does not produce a phosphaturic response. Phenotypically, these patients have mental retardation, shortness of stature, and obesity.

436. The answer is c. (*Behrman, 16/e, pp. 200–201, 1580–1581. McMillan, 3/e, pp. 83–84, 1770–1772. Rudolph, 20/e, pp. 1338, 1844–1847.*) Hypercalcemia can develop in children who are immobilized following the fracture of a weight-bearing bone. Serious complications of immobilization hypercalcemia, and the hypercalciuria that occurs as a result, include nephropathy, nephrocalcinosis, hypertensive encephalopathy, and convulsions. The early symptoms of hypercalcemia—namely, constipation, anorexia, occasional vomiting, polyuria, and lethargy—are nonspecific and may be ascribed to the effects of the injury and hospitalization. Therefore, careful monitoring of these patients with serial measurements of the serum ionized calcium and the urinary calcium–creatinine ratio is critical during their immobilization. A ratio of > 0.2 establishes a diagnosis of hypercalciuria. Although complete mobilization is curative, additional measures such as vigorous intravenous hydration with a balanced salt solution, dietary restrictions of dairy products, and administration of diuretics can be instituted. For patients who are at risk for symptomatic hypercalcemia, short-term therapy with calcitonin is highly effective in reducing the concentration of serum calcium by inhibiting bone resorption.

437. The answer is d. *(Behrman, 16/e, p. 1782. McMillan, 3/e, p. 1797. Rudolph, 20/e, p. 1817.)* Glucose is nonenzymatically attached to hemoglobin to form glycosylated hemoglobin. The major component of this reaction proceeds very slowly and is irreversible until the hemoglobin is destroyed. The concentration of glycosylated hemoglobin thus reflects glucose concentration over the half-life of the red cell, or about 2 to 3 months.

438–439. The answers are 438–b, 439–b. *(Behrman, 16/e, pp. 1729–1736. McMillan, 3/e, pp. 311,1806–1809, 1816–1820. Rudolph, 20/e, pp. 1068, 1683, 1725–1728, 1764, 1765.)* Salt-losing congenital adrenal hyperplasia (adrenogenital syndrome; 21-hydroxylase deficiency) usually manifests during the first 5 to 15 days of life as anorexia, vomiting, diarrhea, and dehydration. Hypoglycemia can also occur. Affected infants can have increased pigmentation, and female infants show evidence of virilization, that is, ambiguous external genitalia. Hyponatremia, hyperkalemia, and urinary sodium wasting are the usual laboratory findings. Death can occur if the diagnosis is missed and appropriate treatment is not instituted. Although adrenal aplasia, an extremely rare disorder, presents a similar clinical picture, it has an earlier onset than adrenal hyperplasia, and virilization does not occur. In classic 21-hydroxylase deficiency, serum levels of 17-hydroxyprogesterone are markedly elevated beyond 3 days of life (in the first 3 days of life they can normally be high). Blood cortisol levels are usually low in salt-losing forms of the disease.

Pyloric stenosis seems unlikely in this infant in that the vomiting with this disease usually begins after the third week of life. Hypothyroidism would present as a lethargic, poor-feeding infant with delayed reflexes, persistent jaundice, and hypotonia. Hyperaldosteronism would be expected to cause decreased potassium, not increased levels. Panhypopituatarism usually presents with apnea, cyanosis, or severe hypoglycemia.

440. The answer is a. *(Behrman, 16/e, p. 349. McMillan, 3/e, pp. 1825, 1829–1830, 1832, 1841–1843. Rudolph, 20/e, pp. 306–311, 313–314, 320.)* The infant described in the question has alkaptonuria, an autosomal recessive disorder caused by a deficiency of homogentisic acid oxidase. The diagnosis is made in infants when their urine turns dark brown or black on exposure to air due to the oxidation of homogentisic acid. Affected children are asymptomatic. In adults, ochronosis—the deposition of a bluish pigment in cartilage and fibrous tissue—develops; symptoms of arthritis may appear later. No specific treatment is available for patients who have alkaptonuria although supplemental ascorbic acid may delay the onset of the disorder and reduce clinical symptoms. The other deficiencies listed in the question are found in phenylketonuria, histidinemia, maple syrup urine disease, and isovaleric acidemia, respectively.

441. The answer is e. *(Behrman, 16/e, pp. 1209–1210. McMillan, 3/e, pp. 1721–1722. Rudolph, 20/e, pp. 369–371.)* Wilson's disease is an autosomal recessive disorder characterized by liver disease, neurologic and behavioral disturbances, renal tubular dysfunction (Fanconi's syndrome), and eye findings. Its multisystem manifestations are caused by the deposition of copper in various tissues (resulting in low serum levels), and therapy is aimed at the prevention of accumulation of copper. Defective metabolism of the copper-binding protein ceruloplasmin (usually reduced) has been demonstrated by some.

442. The answer is d. *(Behrman, 16/e, pp. 1562–1563, 1666, 1729–1739, 1758–1759, 1761–1765. McMillan, 3/e, pp. 351–352, 1533–1535, 1816–1820, 1774. Rudolph, 20/e, pp. 1725–1728, 1731–1735, 1780–1781.)* Patients with testicular feminization are genotypic males with normal testes. Complete resistance to androgens causes failure of masculinization of the external genitalia, which remain female. At puberty, these persons develop normal female breasts and body habitus despite the presence of testes and high concentrations of testosterone. Because of resistance to androgens, these patients have scant secondary sexual hair and, thus, do not develop hirsutism. The other disorders listed represent syndromes of excess androgens and, therefore, can cause hirsutism.

443. The answer is d. *(Behrman, 16/e, pp. 184–187. McMillan, 3/e, pp. 83, 471, 474, 1619, 1900. Rudolph, 20/e, pp. 1839–1840, 1847–1849.)* Nutritional rickets is caused by a dietary deficiency of vitamin D and lack of exposure to sunlight. Intestinal absorption of calcium and phosphorus is diminished in vitamin D deficiency. Transient hypocalcemia stimulates the secretion of parathyroid hormone and the mobilization of calcium and phosphorus from bone; enhanced parathyroid hormone activity leads to phosphaturia and diminished excretion of calcium. In children with nutritional rickets, the concentration of serum calcium usually is normal and the phosphate level low. Increased serum alkaline phosphatase is a common finding. The excretion of calcium in the urine is increased only after therapy with vitamin D has been instituted.

444. The answer is d. *(Behrman, 16/e, pp. 330–332, 1606–1687, 1747 1749, 2131–2132. McMillan, 3/e, pp. 1833–1835, 2231, 2241, 2248. Rudolph, 20/e, pp, 392–394, 400–401, 1785–1786.)* Marfan's syndrome is a genetic disorder transmitted as an autosomal dominant trait with variable expression. People with this disorder usually have tall stature, arachnodactyly, subluxation of the lens, dilatation of the aorta, and dissecting aneurysm. Mental retardation is not a part of this syndrome. Vascular complications are the usual cause of death. Patients with any of the other syndromes listed have tall stature and varying degrees of mental retardation among their clinical findings.

445. The answer is a. *(Behrman, 16/e, pp. 533–534. McMillan, 3/e, p. 208. Rudolph, 20/e, pp. 1831–1832.)* Glycogen and fat stores are diminished in premature infants and those small for gestational age. Energy stores are inadequate to meet the energy demands after the maternal supply of glucose is interrupted at birth, and hypoglycemia ensues. Deficiency of cortisol or growth hormone is a rare cause of neonatal hypoglycemia. Insulin excess, common in infants of diabetic mothers, is unusual in other infants. Hypoglycemia associated with a deficiency of glucagon has been reported but is very rare.

446. The answer is b. (*Behrman, 16/e, pp. 224–227. McMillan, 3/e, pp. 1768–1769. Rudolph, 20/e, pp. 1841–1843.*) Hypocalcemia of newborn infants can be divided into two groups: early (during the first approximately 72 h of life) and late (after approximately 72 h). The most common type of early neonatal hypocalcemia is the so-called idiopathic hypocalcemia. Other causes early on include maternal illness (diabetes, toxemia, and hyperparathyroidism), neonatal respiratory distress (perinatal asphyxia) or sepsis, low birth weight due to prematurity, or hypomagnesemia. Transient or permanent hypoparathyroidism and high phosphate intake are the most common factors associated with late hypocalcemia.

447–451. The answers are 447–a, 448–e, 449–d, 450–b, 451–d. (*Behrman, 16/e, pp. 1713–1714, 1718–1722, 2128–2130, 2136–2137. McMillan, 3/e, pp. 1618–1621, 1770–1772, 1812, 1896–1897. Rudolph, 20/e, pp. 387–389, 1842, 1844–1845, 1847–1849.*) Vitamin D–resistant rickets is caused by a genetic abnormality in the renal tubular reabsorption of phosphate with resultant hyperphosphaturia and hypophosphatemia and also in the conversion of 25-hydroxyvitamin D to 1,25-dihydroxyvitamin D. The intestinal absorption of phosphate is also abnormal and calcium absorption from the gut can be secondarily affected. Calcium concentration is usually normal. The disorder is usually transmitted as an X-linked dominant trait.

Patients with pseudohypoparathyroidism have the same chemical abnormality (low Ca, high PO_4) as those with hypoparathyroidism. They are distinguished from the latter group by the phenotypic features and high serum concentration of parathyroid hormone. The basic abnormality in these patients is the unresponsiveness of the renal tubules to parathyroid hormone. They are classified into two groups depending on the site of the defect. Type I patients have failure to generate cyclic AMP and do not have an increase in urinary concentration of cyclic AMP or phosphate in response to parathyroid hormone. Type II patients have a defect in the renal tubules that causes failure to respond to high concentrations of cyclic AMP. These patients, if given parathyroid hormone, have increased urinary excretion of cyclic AMP but not of phosphate.

Osteogenesis imperfecta is transmitted as an autosomal recessive (severe form) or, more commonly, autosomal dominant (milder form) disorder. The basic defect is an abnormality in the production and composition of the matrix of bone. Serum calcium and phosphate concentrations are normal.

Hyperparathyroidism is rare in children. In response to high concentrations of parathyroid hormone, there is increased bone resorption. In the kidney, there is increased excretion of phosphate and enhanced formation of 1,25-dihydroxyvitamin D. Increased formation of 1,25-dihydroxyvitamin D, in turn, enhances the absorption of calcium and, secondarily, of phosphorus from the gut. The net effect is hypercalcemia and hypophosphatemia.

Medullary carcinoma of thyroid arises from the C cells of the thyroid. These tumors secrete excessive amounts of calcitonin and accordingly, the concentration of this hormone in the blood is increased. Despite elevated levels of calcitonin, the serum concentration of calcium and of phosphorus is usually normal unless the patient has associated hyperparathyroidism (multiple endocrine adenomatosis, type II).

452–457. The answers are 452–e, 453–a, 454–b, 455–e, 456–e, 457–b. (*Behrman, 16/e, pp. 1718–1719, 1737–1739, 1746–1747, 1922. McMillan, 3/e, pp. 1620–1621, 1819–1820, 2246. Rudolph, 20/e, pp. 400, 1731–1734, 1802, 1842, 1988.*) The Prader-Willi syndrome is a disorder consisting of hypotonia, hypogonadism, hyperphagia after the newborn period, hypomentia, and obesity. A deletion of a portion of chromosome 15 has been found in approximately 70 percent of patients. Children affected by this syndrome exhibit little movement in utero and are hypotonic during the neonatal period. Feeding difficulties and failure to thrive can be the presenting complaints in the first year; later, obesity becomes the most common presenting complaint. The enormous food intake of affected children is thought to be due to a defect in the satiety center in the hypothalamus. Stringent caloric restriction is the only known treatment.

Laurence-Moon-Biedl syndrome is transmitted as an autosomal recessive trait. Obesity, mental retardation, hypogonadism, polydactyly, and retinitis pigmentosa with night blindness are the principal findings in affected children. There is no known effective treatment.

The initial complaint in Cushing's syndrome may be obesity. Accumulation of fat in the face, neck, and trunk causes the characteristic "buffalo hump" and "moon" facies. Characteristic features include growth failure, muscle wasting, thinning of the skin, plethora, and hypertension. The bone age of affected patients is retarded, and osteoporosis can be present. The disorder results from an excess of glucocorticoids that may be caused by a primary adrenal abnormality (adenoma or carcinoma) or secondary hypercortisolism, which may be due to excess adrenocorticotropin. Exogenous glucocorticoids administered in supraphysiologic doses for a prolonged period of time will produce a similar picture in normal subjects.

Pseudohypoparathyroidism is a collective term for a variety of diseases. Affected patients have biochemical findings (low serum calcium and high serum phosphorus levels) similar to those associated with hypoparathyroidism, but they also have high levels of endogenous parathyroid hormone; in addition, exogenous parathyroid hormone fails to increase their phosphate excretion or raise their serum calcium level. The defects in these patients appear to be at the hormone receptor site or in the adenylate cyclase-cyclic AMP system. The symptoms of pseudohypoparathyroidism are due to hypocalcemia. Affected children are short, round-faced, and mildly retarded. Metacarpals and metatarsals are shortened, and subcutaneous and basal ganglia calcifications as well as cataracts can be present. The current treatment consists of large doses of vitamin D and reduction of the phosphate load.

Fröhlich's syndrome has none of the characteristics listed in the question.

458–463. The answers are 458–a, 459–e, 460–e, 461–d, 462–a, 463–b. *(Behrman, 16/e, pp. 195–196, 408–409, 1600–1601, 1726, 1729–1736, 1739–1740. McMillan, 3/e, pp. 1621–1624, 1792, 1813, 1816–1819, 1855–1856. Rudolph, 20/e, pp. 330–331, 1705–1708, 1725–1730, 1735.)* In the salt-losing variety of 21-hydroxylase deficiency, the synthesis of both mineralocorticoids (e.g., aldosterone) and cortisol is impaired. Aldosterone deficiency impairs the exchange of potassium for sodium in the distal renal tubule. Affected patients have hyponatremia and hyperkalemia. Dehydration, hypotension, and shock may be present.

In the absence of vasopressin, renal collecting tubules are impermeable to water, resulting in the excretion of hypotonic urine. Patients with diabetes insipidus present with polyuria and polydipsia. Net loss of water leads to dehydration and hemoconcentration and, therefore, to relatively high serum concentrations of sodium and potassium. Patients with nephrogenic diabetes insipidus have similar laboratory findings. This genetic disorder is unresponsive to antidiuretic hormone (ADH). These patients are unable to concentrate their urine and present in the neonatal period with hypernatremic dehydration.

In hyperaldosteronism, renal tubular sodium–potassium exchange is enhanced. Hypokalemia, hypernatremia, hyperchloremia, and alkalosis are the usual findings. Primary hyperaldosteronism (Conn's syndrome) is very rare in children.

Addison's disease is associated with a combined deficiency of glucocorticoids and mineralocorticoids. Resorption of sodium and excretion of potassium and hydrogen ions are impaired at the level of the distal renal tubules. Sodium loss results in loss of water and depletion of blood volume. Persons with compensated Addison's disease can have relatively normal physical and laboratory findings; addisonian crisis, however, characteristically produces hyponatremia, hyperkalemia, and shock. The pathophysiology of the serum electrolyte abnormalities in this disorder is the same as in the salt-losing variety of adrenogenital syndrome.

Patients with a deficiency of glucose-6-phosphatase (von Gierke's disease) are, as a rule, hyperlipidemic. Increased triglyceride concentration in the serum decreases the volume of the aqueous compartment. Because electrolytes are present only in the aqueous compartment of the serum but are expressed in milliequivalents per liter of serum as a whole, the concentrations of sodium and potassium can be facutiously low in these patients.

464–468. The answers are 464–c, 465–h, 466–e, 467–b, 468–a. (*Behrman, 16/e, pp. 713–716, 1588–1589, 1599–1600, 2134. McMillan, 3/e, pp. 1545–1546, 1615–1616, 1618–1620, 1882–1883, 2162–2165. Rudolph, 20/e, pp. 486–489, 909, 1350–1351, 1381, 1848–1849.*) All the disorders listed in the question are familial, even systemic lupus erythematosus, which appears to result from a combination of environmental and genetic causes. Lupus has been postulated to result from sun, drugs, or infection in genetically predisposed persons.

Hypophosphatemic rickets (vitamin D–resistant rickets) is usually inherited as an X-linked dominant trait. Affected males, therefore, have a more severe form of this disease than affected females. Variants of the classic form also seem to be transmitted on occasion as an autosomal recessive and even as an autosomal dominant trait.

Polycystic kidney and liver disease is an autosomal recessive disorder that is associated with the development of hepatic fibrosis as children get older. Renal failure can occur early in infancy but is of variable severity. It can lead to the need for dialysis and renal transplant. Liver disease, the main source of later problems, can lead to portal hypertension.

Adult-type polycystic kidney disease, inherited in an autosomal dominant fashion, is often seen in successive generations of the same family.

If adult-type polycystic kidney disease is discovered, the family requires investigation.

Cystinosis is an autosomal recessive disease in which affected patients can develop renal failure in childhood or adolescence, or a more benign form in which renal failure does not occur; however, crystalline deposits in cornea can occur. Now that some patients who have cystine storage disease are receiving renal allografts, the pathologic effects of cystine storage in tissues other than the kidney may become clinically important.

469–470. The answers are 469–a, 470–c. (*Behrman, 16/e, pp. 331, 1746–1747, 1884–1885. McMillan, 3/e, pp. 1979–1981, 2234, 2246. Rudolph, 20/e, pp. 305–306, 400, 1988, 2034–2039.*) The mitochondrial genome originates only from the ovum and is, therefore, transmitted by the mother to her offspring of both sexes. Mitochondrial disease involves mainly brain and muscle. Ragged red fibers seen on muscle biopsy are seen in several inherited enzyme defects. Examples of mitochondrial inheritance include myoclonic epilepsy and ragged red fibers (MERF); mitochondrial myopathy, encephalopathy, lactic acidosis, and stroke-like episodes (MELAS); and Leber's hereditary optic neuropathy (LHON), a condition not associated with myopathy. Prader-Willi syndrome, which is characterized by hypotonia, obesity, hypogonadism, mental retardation, and characteristic hands, feet, and facies, is caused by a chromosomal deletion of 15q11-13 when the chromosome is of paternal origin. Chromosomal deletion of maternal origin results in Angelman's syndrome, characterized by a specific facies, happy disposition, mental retardation, bizarre movements, and seizures. More recently, cases of Prader-Willi syndrome have been found wherein there is no DNA deletion but both copies of chromosome 15 have been inherited from the mother; similarly, some cases of Angelman's syndrome have been shown to have two copies of paternally derived chromosome 15. This suggests that it is the lack of part of paternal chromosome 15 that causes Prader-Willi syndrome and lack of part of maternal chromosome 15 that causes Angelman's syndrome.

471–472. The answers are 471–a, 472–d. (*Behrman, 16/e, pp. 52–57. McMillan, 3/e, pp. 527–530. Rudolph, 20/e, p. 1794.*) The first sign of pubertal changes in girls is the development of breast buds (as early as 8 years). In boys, testicular enlargement occurs first, often as early as 9.5 years. Pubertal changes then follow a rather set sequence commonly known as Tanner staging. Normal ranges for the various levels of development of secondary sexual characteristics are available.

473–474. The answers are 473–b, c, f; 474–c, i, l. *(Behrman, 16/e, pp. 328, 330, 1753–1755. McMillan, 3/e, pp. 2230–2231. Rudolph, 20/e, pp. 297–299, 1782–1784.)* Common features of Turner's syndrome include female phenotype, short stature, sexual infantilism, streak gonads, broad chest, low hairline, webbed neck, congenital lymphedema of the hands and feet, coarctation of the aorta, and a variety of other anomalies.

Down syndrome has many diagnostic features including short stature, microcephaly, centrally placed hair whorl, small ears, redundant skin on the nape of the neck, upslanting palpebral fissures, epicanthal folds, flat nasal bridge, Brushfield's spots, protruding tongue, short and broad hands, simian creases, widely spaced first and second toe, and hypotonia. Cardiac lesions are found in 30 percent to 50 percent of children with Down syndrome, including endocardial cushion defect (30 percent), ventricular septal defect (30 percent), and tetralogy of Fallot (about 30 percent). At birth, duodenal atresia is a common finding. It causes bilious vomiting and a characteristic KUB finding of a double bubble (dilatation of the stomach and the proximal duodenum)

THE ADOLESCENT

Questions

DIRECTIONS: Each item below contains a question or incomplete statement followed by suggested responses. Select the **one best** response to each question.

475. In evaluating an adolescent, the examiner looks for evidence of healthy mental development. Which of the following manifestations of mid-adolescence should raise concern?

a. close, enduring friendships with peers of the same gender
b. rejection of parental standards and beliefs, such as those regarding religion or sexual conduct
c. disregard for physical well-being
d. concern for weight and body configuration
e. frequent bickering and quarreling with siblings

476. In evaluating an adolescent, which of the following should be considered normal?

a. involvement in extracurricular activities or a job to the detriment of schoolwork
b. absence of aims or plans for the near or far future
c. changing and fleeting romantic attachments (lasting 3 months or less) or multiple simultaneous attachments
d. preoccupation with physical well-being; concern for physical symptoms
e. constant bickering and quarreling with friends

477. A 15-year-old boy has been advised by his athletic coach to begin a course of anabolic steroids. He asks you to write a prescription. Potential toxic effects of the anabolic steroids include which of the following?

a. hypoglycemia
b. increased testicular size
c. increased high-density lipoproteins
d. toxic hepatitis
e. delayed closure of epiphyses

478. A 15-year-old girl is brought to the pediatric emergency room by the lunchroom teacher, who observed her sitting alone and crying. On questioning, the teacher learned that the girl had taken five tablets after having had an argument with her mother about a boyfriend of whom the mother disapproved. Toxicology studies are negative and physical examination is normal. The most appropriate course of action would be to

a. hospitalize the teenager on the adolescent ward
b. get a psychiatry consultation
c. get a social service consultation
d. arrange a family conference that includes the boyfriend
e. prescribe an antidepressant and arrange for a prompt clinic appointment

479. Which of the following statements applicable to anorexia nervosa or bulimia is correct?

a. rarely do anorexia and bulimia occur in the same patient simultaneously

b. anorexia nervosa most commonly occurs in girls less than 10 years old

c. no signs of bulimia can be found on careful physical examination

d. when used appropriately, imipramine is a useful adjunct in the treatment of bulimia

e. girls with anorexia nervosa are usually too weak to engage in active sports

480. A 17-year-old sexually active girl comes to your office complaining of acne unresponsive to the usual treatment regimen. Physical examination reveals severe nodulocystic acne of her face and upper chest and back. You consider prescribing isotretinoin (Accutane), but you are concerned about side effects. Reviewing the literature, you find which of the following to be true about isotretinoin?

a. its efficacy can be profound and permanent

b. it is not known to be a teratogen

c. most patients experience excessive tearing and salivation

d. severe arthritis necessitating cessation of the drug occurs in about 15 percent of patients

e. significant decrease in serum triglyceride levels are noted in 25 percent of patients

481. A 15-year-old presents with the complaint of a rash as pictured. Which of the following statements is correct concerning the management of this common condition?

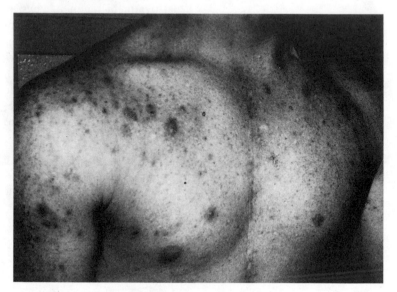

(Courtesy Adelaide Hebert, M.D.)

a. fried foods must be avoided
b. frequent scrubbing of the face is key
c. topical antibiotics are of no value
d. topical benzoyl peroxide is the mainstay of treatment
e. this rash is solely a disease of the adolescent

482. Concerning adolescent suicide, which of the following statements is true?

a. girls tend to use more lethal means
b. the number of attempted suicides is much higher in boys
c. most suicide attempters and completers (where a history can be established) have a history of a prior attempt or prior serious suicidal ideation
d. inquiry by pediatricians about suicidal thoughts precipitates the act
e. the number of suicides in adolescents 10 to 19 years of age decreased significantly since the 1950s and is now a rare cause of death in adolescents

483. For which age group of females is idiopathic scoliosis the most common?

a. birth to 3 years
b. 4 to 10 years
c. 11 to 18 years
d. 19 to 25 years

484. Warning signs of drug or alcohol abuse include which of the following?

a. excessive concern for weight and body configuration
b. improved school performance
c. recent changes from age-appropriate, acceptable friends to younger associates
d. deterioration in personal habits, hygiene, dress, grooming, speech patterns, and fluency of expression
e. improvement in relationships with adults, siblings, and authority figures

485. Teenage pregnancies and their complications are an increasing problem that calls for a comprehensive approach. In teenage pregnancy there is

a. an increased risk of pre-eclampsia and eclampsia
b. a higher rate of post-date delivery
c. reduced incidence of infant mortality
d. an increased risk of large for gestation age infants
e. a higher probability of multiple births

486. A 15-year-old boy asks how to bulk up. Appropriate advice to increase muscle mass includes

a. taking extra vitamins
b. doubling protein intake
c. using hormones
d. increasing muscle work
e. taking ergogenic medication

487. A 15-year-old sexually active girl is seen in an adolescent clinic for her yearly checkup. Appropriate screening tests for sexually transmitted diseases should be part of that visit. Which of the following sexually transmitted diseases can be diagnosed only when the patient is symptomatic?

a. endocervical culture for *Neisseria gonorrhoeae*
b. endocervical culture or antigen test for *Chlamydia trachomatis*
c. Papanicolaou (Pap) smear
d. test for herpes simplex type 2
e. serologic test for syphilis

488. An 18-year-old male college student is seen in the student health clinic for urinary frequency, dysuria, and urethral discharge. Which of the following is LEAST likely to be encountered in the evaluation of this man?

a. gonorrhea
b. chlamydial urethritis
c. *Esherichia coli* urinary tract infection
d. syphilis
e. HIV infection

489. A 19-year-old male college student returns from spring break in Fort Lauderdale, Florida, with complaints of acute pain and swelling of the scrotum. Which of the following is LEAST likely to be the cause of his problem?

a. epididymitis
b. torsion of testicle
c. trauma to testicle
d. urinary stones
e. strangulated inguinal hernia

Items 490–491

490. A 16-year-old girl presents with lower abdominal pain and fever. On physical examination, a tender adnexal mass is felt. Further questioning in private reveals the following: she has a new sexual partner; her periods are irregular; she has a vaginal discharge. The LEAST likely diagnosis is

a. appendiceal abscess
b. tuboovarian abscess
c. ovarian cyst
d. renal cyst
e. ectopic pregnancy

491. You hospitalize the patient for closely supervised treatment. In addition to the acute complications, there are possible long-term sequelae. These include which of the following?

a. ectopic pregnancy
b. increased incidence of twining
c. chronic fatigue syndrome
d. ovarian cancer
e. endometriosis

DIRECTIONS: Each group of questions below consists of lettered options followed by numbered items. For each numbered item, select the appropriate lettered option(s). Each lettered option may be used once, more than once, or not at all. **Choose exactly the number of options indicated following each item.**

Items 492–495

Listed below are diseases in which genital ulcers may occur. Match each with the appropriate diagnostic test.

a. dark-field microscopic examination
b. special chocolate agar culture
c. Bordet-Gengou medium culture
d. Tzanck preparation for multinucleated giant cells
e. *Chlamydia* culture
f. Loeffler medium culture

492. Syphilis
(SELECT 1 TEST)

493. Herpes simplex
(SELECT 1 TEST)

494. Lymphogranuloma venereum
(SELECT 1 TEST)

495. Chancroid
(SELECT 1 TEST)

Items 496–500

Listed below are common injuries of the adolescent. Match each with the activity with which it is most commonly associated.

a. swimming
b. football
c. basketball
d. running
e. ballet
f. wrestling
g. skiing
h. hockey

496. Patellar tendinitis and Osgood-Schlatter disease
(SELECT 1 ACTIVITY)

497. Injuries almost exclusively related to the shoulder, including rotator cuff tendinitis
(SELECT 1 ACTIVITY)

498. Delayed menarche and eating disorder
(SELECT 1 ACTIVITY)

499. Hyperextension of the thumb and sprains of the anterior cruciate ligament
(SELECT 1 ACTIVITY)

500. Shoulder subluxation, knee injuries, and dermatologic problems such as herpes simplex, impetigo, and staphylococcal furunculosis or folliculitis
(SELECT 1 ACTIVITY)

THE ADOLESCENT

Answers

475–476. The answers are 475–c, 476–c. *(Behrman, 16/e, pp. 52–57. McMillan, 3/e, pp. 531–536. Rudolph, 20/e, pp. 39–45.)* Adolescence is a time of major physical, cognitive, and emotional changes. The tasks of the adolescent are directed toward determining his or her ultimate adult self. He or she must become independent of his or her parents and in so doing, take responsibility for his or her own welfare and start preparing for his or her future work or career. He or she must define himself or herself sexually and move toward lasting attachments. The range of normality is broad and the variations numerous. Evaluation of the adolescent requires weighing the normal and abnormal tendencies to determine where the balance lies. To neglect schoolwork and have no vision or plan for the future suggests either immaturity or depression. A certain degree of concern for appearance is a healthy adolescent phenomenon. On the other hand, excessive concern for physical well-being and physical symptoms suggests an abnormal level of anxiety or depression. Constant quarreling with friends indicates a lack of flexibility and accommodation. Close friends help in the separation from parents and the achievement of independence by providing mutual support and self-justification. Bickering with siblings, on the other hand, is a holdover from childhood and, if not excessive, may be considered normal. Brief superficial romantic attractions fueled more by fantasy than reality start in early to mid-adolescence. These are rehearsals for the more serious attachments to come.

477. The answer is d. *(Behrman, 16/e, pp. 571–572. McMillan, 3/e, p. 1774. Rudolph, 20/e, pp. 1795–1796.)* As his physician, you point out the untoward medical consequences, which include decrease in testicular size, oligospermia, aggressive behavior, mood swings, liver damage, and decreased levels of high-density lipoproteins, as well as possible premature closure of epiphyses. In addition, you point out that the use of anabolic steroids may give the athlete an unfair advantage and, therefore, using them is tantamount to cheating.

478. The answer is a. *(Behrman, 16/e, pp. 559–560. McMillan, 3/e, pp. 810–812. Rudolph, 20/e, pp. 172–173.)* The adolescent who has attempted suicide should be hospitalized so that a complete medical, psychological, and social evaluation can be performed and an appropriate treatment plan developed. Hospitalization also emphasizes the seriousness of the adolescent's action to her and to her family and the importance of cooperation in carrying out the recommendations for ongoing future therapy. The treatment plan may include continued counseling or supportive therapy with a pediatrician, outpatient psychotherapy with a psychiatrist or other mental health worker, or family therapy.

479. The answer is d. *(Behrman, 16/e, pp. 562–564. McMillan, 3/e, pp. 651, 813–820. Rudolph, 20/e, pp. 43–44.)* Eating disorders have become increasingly prevalent in recent years. Symptoms of finicky appetite, progressively restricted food intake, distress at looking fat, and compulsively pursuing thinness can appear after puberty. Parents may not appreciate the magnitude of weight loss until it reaches 10 percent or more of body weight because those girls will not undress in their parents' presence and because the facial contours are the last parts to be affected. Bulimia usually appears in mid-adolescence rather than early adolescence and is characterized by sessions of gorging, often in secret and often involving a single favored snack food such as ice cream, cake, or candy, although it may also be manifested as immoderate eating at mealtimes. This gorging is followed by secret bouts of self-induced vomiting. Some bulimics also use laxatives and purgatives. Physical consequences of bulimia include esophageal varices and hemorrhage; dental decay, especially of anterior teeth (because of exposure of enamel to HCl); and a swollen, reddened, irritated uvula (also from chronic HCl exposure). Physical consequences of anorexia include profound weight loss (25 percent to 30 percent or more of body weight), dehydration, facial and arm hirsutism, loss of hair of the head, bradycardia, cardiac conduction problems, hypocardia, hypothermia, impaired renal function, multiple malnutrition effects (including avitaminoses), a primary or secondary amenorrhea, and osteoporosis. There is significant mortality in treatment-resistant cases. The psychological component of these disorders is not a unitary one. Some anorexic patients have an underlying obsessive-compulsive or narcissistic personality disorder, some are borderline psychotic, and some are depressed. Bulimic patients have a significant underlying depression. Patients with eating disorders have exceedingly ambivalent feelings toward parents, especially mothers, and in turn evoke great ambivalence on the part of parents. Therapy includes behavior modification to deal with eating behavior per se, family therapy, and individual or group therapy. Imipramine, when used appropriately, is a useful adjunct treatment for this condition. In cases of life-threatening degrees of weight loss or vomiting, hospitalization to limit freedom, restore physiologic equilibrium, and provide a controlled eating environment can be indicated.

480. The answer is a. (*Behrman, 16/e, pp. 2047–2049. McMillan, 3/e, pp. 729–731, 2229. Rudolph, 20/e, pp. 924–925.*) Isotretinoin (13-*cis*-retinoic acid; Accutane) has proved to be very effective in the treatment of refractory nodulocystic acne. The effects of treatment appear to be long lasting. Precautions regarding its use, however, are essential. Because of its teratogenic effects (isotretinoin syndrome), the drug is contraindicated during pregnancy and within 1 month of becoming pregnant. Dry skin, eyes, and mucous membranes are the most frequent complications of therapy. Other associated problems include musculoskeletal pain and hyperostosis, inflammatory bowel disease, pseudotumor cerebri, and corneal opacities. Patients on isotretinoin therapy can often develop abnormal liver function tests, elevated triglyceride and cholesterol levels, and lowered levels of high-density lipoproteins.

481. The answer is d. (*Behrman, 16/e, pp. 2047–2049. McMillan, 3/e, pp. 729–731. Rudolph, 20/e, pp. 924–925.*) Acne is a skin disorder that affects virtually all adolescents and is seen less commonly in older patients. There is a wide spectrum of clinical findings ranging from a few papules and comedones to a disfiguring nodulocystic disease of the face and trunk. The goals of therapy are to prevent scarring and disfigurement and to avoid loss of self-esteem. The chief benefit of benzoyl peroxide is derived from its antibacterial activity, but it also functions as an exfoliant and comedolytic. A combination of benzoyl peroxide and retinoic acid is particularly effective in sloughing the epithelium, and statics, such as oral tetracycline, and the use of topical antibiotics can be necessary to control the inflammatory component of acne. Studies have failed to demonstrate adverse effects of any particular foods on disease activity. Vigorous facial scrubbing can traumatize the skin and aggravate the problem.

482. The answer is c. *(Behrman, 16/e, pp. 599–560. McMillan, 3/e, pp. 810–812. Rudolph, 20/e, pp. 27, 172–173.)* Suicide among teenagers has increased steadily since 1950 and is now the third leading cause of adolescent death, following accidents and homicides. Suicide attempts occur more often in girls, but in all age groups, males outnumber females in completed suicides because boys tend to use more lethal means, such as firearms, hanging, jumping, and inhalation of carbon monoxide. Most suicide attempters and completers (where history can be established) have a history of a prior attempt or prior serious suicidal ideation. Therefore, direct questioning of the adolescent about feelings of sadness, hopelessness, concerns about death, and thoughts of committing suicide is important. There are no data to indicate that such inquiry precipitates suicidal behavior.

483. The answer is c. *(Behrman, 16/e, pp. 2083–2084. McMillan, 3/e, pp. 2117–2121. Rudolph, 20/e, pp. 2153–2155.)* The most common form of scoliosis is idiopathic scoliosis. Three age ranges of idiopathic scoliosis exist: infantile (which presents at birth to 3 years of age), juvenile (presenting at 4 to 10 years of age), and adolescent (the most common form, accounting for 80 percent of cases and presenting from 11 years and older). To diagnose this condition, the back is viewed from behind with the patient in the standing position. The waist, shoulders, and pelvis should be symmetric. The spine is examined for symmetry or deformity. The patient is then asked to bring the palms together in the front and bend at the waist. Viewing the patient from behind will allow for identification of any humps, valleys, or other deformities of the spine. Identified abnormalities can be confirmed radiographically. Premenarchal girls with a curvature of the spine of more than 20 degrees on radiographs need close follow-up every 4 to 6 months because the risk of progression is high.

484. The answer is d. *(Behrman, 16/e, pp. 564–567. McMillan, 3/e, pp. 550–555. Rudolph, 20/e, pp. 807–808.)* When an adolescent shows evidence of declining school performance or truancy, a change for the worse in personal habits and grooming, exaggerated mood swings, change in friends to an older and unacceptable group of friends, and frequent hostile reactions in relationships with others, the possibility that he or she is abusing drugs or alcohol or both should be strongly considered. Dependence on drugs is a progressive disorder; therefore, prompt identification and intervention are required if serious complications are to be avoided. Routine health assessment of adolescents should include inquiry about the use of cigarettes, alcohol, and other drugs, and about school performance and family and peer relationships.

485. The answer is a. *(Behrman, 16/e, pp. 580–582. McMillan, 3/e, p. 543.)* The main obstetric complications of teenage pregnancy are preeclampsia and eclampsia, which are thought to be due to inadequate prenatal care and nutrition. The rate of prematurity is high, and this in turn is thought to account for the increased incidence of mental retardation among children of teenage mothers. The incidence of repeat pregnancy and infant mortality is high. A combination of medical, social, psychological, and educational resources must be made available to permit optimum health and development of the teenage mother and her child. Multiple births do not occur with any greater frequency in teenagers than in older women.

486. The answer is d. *(Behrman, 16/e, p. 2110. McMillan, 3/e, p. 736. Rudolph, 20/e, pp. 2130–2131.)* Increased muscle work (along with increased calories) is the only appropriate way to increase muscle mass. Measurements of skin-fold thickness, performed serially, are a useful way to detect changes in the amount of body fat, so that obesity can be avoided. Protein loading or using drugs, hormones, and vitamins will not be helpful and may be harmful.

487. The answer is d. *(Behrman, 16/e, pp. 583–586. McMillan, 3/e, pp. 555–559. Rudolph, 20/e, pp. 67–77.)* The sexually active teenager can be screened for all the conditions listed except asymptomatic genital herpes, for which there is no satisfactory screen. A Pap smear can reveal cellular changes that represent precursors of cervical neoplastic disease. Squamous intraepithelial lesions, formerly known as cervical intraepithelial neoplasia (CIN), affect about 5 percent to 10 percent of sexually active adolescents. Gonorrhea can be asymptomatic; syphilis is on the rise; chlamydial infection is present in 10 percent to 25 percent of all sexually active adolescents. Screening tests for these diseases are readily available. A wet mount of vaginal secretions can demonstrate trichomonal, candidal, and bacterial vaginosis.

488. The answer is c. *(Behrman, 16/e, pp. 583–586. McMillan, 3/e, p. 562. Rudolph, 20/e, pp. 67–73.)* Urethritis in an adolescent male is almost always a sexually transmitted disease (STD), either gonococcal or nongonococcal urethritis (NGU). *Chlamydia trachomatis* is usually the causative agent in NGU. Less frequently, NGU can be caused by *Ureaplasma urealyticum*, *Trichomonas vaginalis*, herpes simplex, and yeast. Gonococcal culture and Gram's stain are easily available; chlamydial culture may not be. Direct monoclonal antibody tests as well as enzyme immunoassay and molecular probe tests are alternative methods for *Chlamydia* identification, although they are less sensitive and less specific than chlamydial culture. Ceftriaxone and doxycycline (among other antibiotics) would be reasonable choices as treatment of urethritis since both gonococcal and nongonococcal infections are covered by these antibiotics. Azithromycin, which has the advantage of a one-dose regimen, may be used instead of doxycycline. Serologic testing for syphilis should always be done. Testing for HIV should be offered and safe sexual practices encouraged. Urinary tract infection is not associated with a urethral discharge.

489. The answer is d. (*Behrman, 16/e, pp. 583–586, 1652–1653. McMillan, 3/e, pp. 1555–1558, 1628–1629. Rudolph, 20/e, pp. 1404–1406.*) Distal ureteral stones can cause pain that is referred to the testes but without local swelling. The most likely diagnosis in this age group, with a possible antecedent history of sexual activity or urinary tract infection, is epididymitis. Causative organisms include *Neisseria gonorrhoeae*, *Chlamydia trachomatis*, and other bacteria. Treatment with appropriate antibiotics and rest are indicated. Testicular torsion, though much less likely to occur in this age group than in younger boys, must always be considered. A radionuclide scan will show diminished uptake in torsion and increased uptake in epididymitis. Doppler ultrasound will demonstrate absence of flow in torsion and increased flow in epididymitis. Prehn's sign, although not totally reliable, is elicited by gently lifting the scrotum toward the symphysis. Relief of the pain points to epididymitis, its worsening to torsion. Strangulated hernia is associated with evidence of intestinal obstruction.

490–491. The answers are 490–d, 491–a. (*Behrman, 16/e, pp. 583–586, 829–832, 919–920. McMillan, 3/e, pp. 561–562. Rudolph, 20/e, pp. 75–76.*) Each year, a diagnosis of pelvic inflammatory disease (PID) is made in over 1 million women. Sexually active teenagers are at great risk of acquiring PID because of their high-risk behavior, exposure to multiple partners, and failure to use contraceptives. The strong likelihood of PID in the patient presented should not preclude consideration of serious conditions requiring surgical intervention, such as appendiceal abscess, tuboovarian abscess, ectopic pregnancy, and ovarian cyst. Renal cyst does not present in the manner described. An episode of PID raises the risk of ectopic pregnancy, and about 20 percent of women become infertile following one episode of PID. Other sequelae include dyspareunia, pyosalpinx, tuboovarian abscess, and pelvic adhesions. Endometriosis is not related to PID.

492–495. The answers are 492–a, 493–d, 494–e, 495–b. *(Behrman, 16/e, pp. 584–585, 838, 903–906, 920, 966–972. McMillan, 3/e, pp. 558–560, 1024–1025, 1120–1121. Rudolph, 20/e, pp. 563–564, 609–610, 654, 883.)* A scraping from a genital ulcer should be examined under dark-field microscopy for *Treponema pallidum*. A serologic test for syphilis is indicated for every sexually active patient recently infected with a sexually transmitted disease. In the event of a negative result, consideration should be given to repeating this test at a later date because serologic tests performed too early in the disease may not be reliable.

A herpes simplex ulcer can be either a primary or a secondary infection. Examination of a Tzanck preparation of scraping from the ulcer reveals multinucleated giant cells and intranuclear inclusions. Herpes simplex virus is readily cultured.

Chancroid caused by *Haemophilus ducreyi* is difficult to culture. Special chocolate agar medium is only 65 percent sensitive. Inguinal adenopathy that suppurates and causes chronic draining of sinuses is commonly seen in chancroid and can be confused with lymphogranuloma venereum (LGV). LGV is caused by serovars of *Chlamydia trachomatis*, which can be cultured. Serial serologic testing for chlamydial antibodies can be of diagnostic value retrospectively.

Genital ulcers probably play a role in the transmission of HIV infection. Moreover, manifestations of syphilis, herpes simplex, and chancroid can be more severe in HIV patients and may not respond as well to standard treatments.

496–500. The answers are 496–c, 497–a, 498–e, 499–g, 500–f. *(Behrman, 16/e, pp. 2110–2112. McMillan, 3/e, pp, 736–737, 742, 745–746, 748. Rudolph, 20/e, pp. 43–44, 2145, 2148.)* A wide variety of injuries occur in adolescents who participate in sports. Some injuries, however, are more common in some sports than in others.

For swimmers, shoulder injuries are the most common type of problem seen. Rotator cuff tendinitis of the biceps and/or the supraspinatus muscles presents as shoulder pain and tenderness.

In football, head and neck injuries are not uncommon, but fortunately serious injuries are rare. Knee injuries such as anterior cruciate, posterior cruciate, and collateral ligament tears do occur. In addition, turf toe, injury to the first metatarsophalangeal joint, is seen when play is on artificial turf.

Basketball and volleyball tend to produce lower extremity problems including the knee with such injuries as Osgood-Schlatter disease and sprains to the ligaments of the knee. Ankle injuries, too, are quite common in these sports.

Injuries due to running are frequently muscle strains in the hamstrings, adductors, soleus, and gastrocnemius muscles. Runner's knee, anterior knee pain due to patellofemoral stress, is also seen.

Ballet can be associated with delayed menarche and eating disorders (more commonly in the female dancers). In addition, a variety of mostly lower extremity problems can be seen ranging from bunions to serious overuse knee and ankle problems. Injuries in wrestlers are frequently seen in the upper extremities, especially shoulder subluxation, and in the knees, usually prepatellar bursitis from traumatic impact to the floor. Additionally, a variety of skin conditions are common ranging from contact dermatitis and superficial fungal infections to herpes simplex (herpes gladiatorum), impetigo, and staphylococcus furunculosis or folliculitis.

Availability of better equipment has resulted in a decrease in the number of serious skiing injuries. Thumb injuries during a fall, skier's thumb (abduction and hyperextension of the thumb causing a sprain of the ulnar collateral ligament), remains the most common injury seen.

Hockey injuries range from mild contusions to significant lacerations. No particular type of injury (with the exception of, perhaps, loss of teeth) is characteristic of this sport.

BIBLIOGRAPHY

Behrman RE, Kliegman RM, Jenson HB. *Nelson Textbook of Pediatrics*, 16/e. Philadelphia: Saunders; 2000.

McMillan JA, DeAngelis CD, Feigin RD, Warshaw JB. *Principles and Practice of Pediatrics*, 3/e. Philadelphia: Lippincott; 1999.

Rudolph AM, Hoffman JIE, Rudolph CD: *Rudolph Pediatrics*, 20/e. Stamford, CT: Appleton & Lange; 1996.

ISBN 0-07-135955-9

90000

9 780071 359559